Brian Door qualified as a_____
Carrington in 1972 and _____
became responsible for running a course in Alexander
Technique for Drama students at Guildhall School of Music
and Drama, the first time such a course had been run there.
Since then he has also run courses in London, New College
Durham, at the University of Newcastle upon Tyne and at
the University of Birmingham, and founded the ongoing
course at DeMontfort University.

In 1979 he started to train teachers, which he has
continued to do ever since. This course is four years long,
taught in Birmingham, and is the only course in the country
examined in all aspects by both written and practical
exams and course work.

Brian Door is the principal director of training course for
the Professional Association of Alexander Teachers. He
lives in Staffordshire with his wife and son.

TOWARDS PERFECT POSTURE

BRIAN DOOR

ORION

An Orion Paperback
First published in Great Britain in 2003 by
Orion Books Ltd,
Orion House, 5 Upper St Martin's Lane,
London WC2H 9EA

A CIP catalogue record for this book
is available from the British Library.

ISBN: 0 75281 680 2

Printed and bound in Great Britain by
Clays Ltd, St Ives plc

To
Leo and Victoria

CONTENTS

ACKNOWLEDGEMENTS
AND THANKS

I begin by acknowledging the gift of life, which I owe to my mum and dad, Charlie and Win, both now dead many years.

It was Roderick Beesley who first told me about the Technique in 1967. He joined Walter Carrington's training course and through him I met two of his fellow students, Ed and Linda Avak, who persuaded me to have lessons.

I want to take this opportunity to recognise my debt to F. M. Alexander who discovered the principles of the Technique round about 1894 and then spent the next sixty years teaching them to whoever he could. Alexander had been dead twelve years before I ever heard of the Alexander Technique so my personal debt to him is the four books he wrote: *Man's Supreme Inheritance*, *Constructive Conscious Control*, *The Use of the Self*, *Universal Constant in Living* – all still in print. Perhaps a bit hard to read now, they come from a different age, but each has large deposits of pure gold. No Alexander teacher could be without them.

Dilys Carrington suggested that I moved in 'above the shop' and I lived there rent-free for years. Peggy Williams paid two terms fees for me when I was behind. My professional debt to Walter Carrington is infinite. I have been practising the Technique, studying Alexander's books and teaching, for thirty years and training teachers for over twenty of them. Each day confirms how faithfully Walter taught me the Technique that he had learned from Alexander. No doubt we would not see eye to eye on everything, but I think we are in absolute agreement about fundamentals. Whilst having his own way of teaching, as we all have, he has not tried to turn the Alexander Technique into the Carrington Technique. Without his fidelity I doubt that there would be an Alexander Technique today. I am steadfastly of his 'school', even though we belong to different professional organisations.

In the progress of my professional life I acknowledge the help, support and friendship of John James, James Dodding, David Gale, Sonja Nerdrum, my singing teacher the late Eduardo Asquez, Allen Percival in London, Nigel Harrison, the late Professor Dennis Matthews in Newcastle, Alan Forde in Durham, the late Jocelyn Powell in Birmingham, Gideon Avrami, Jayne Stevens, Sue Davis in Leicester. I apologise to those whom I may have inadvertently left out. I also apologise if I embarrass those with whom my relationship has been that of supportive friendship, but I must mention some of them. The Holland family, especially Mary, who were so important to me in my student and early teaching years. I would also like to mention Pam Bygate in Newcastle, Brian Bate, Josephine Bird and the late John Roper, in Shrewsbury. Our life-long friends Bob and Toddy Snoding, our friends Clare and David Wilkinson and my four sisters Joan, Connie, Christine and Janet (their husbands and children as well, of course). Most supportive of all, my wife and son.

I am indebted to my colleagues and students and really should mention them all. They will understand, though, if I mention only my co-directors of Training Course, Kevin Edwards, Martin Leach, Dorothy Burnicle; our assistants Joanna Walker, Rose Whyman, Ian Whaley, Priscilla Hebblethwaite, all of whom are also friends. Lastly my friend and colleague, to whom I first gave lessons twenty-seven years ago, Fred Oldfield, who is the mainstay of us all.

I want to mention Doreen Montgomery of Rupert Crewe, through whose agency I got this commission and who has looked after me so well. Also, I want to thank my two editors at Orion Publishing, Caroline Oakley and Juliet Ewers, for everything.

What this book is about and how it can help you

We all want to enjoy good health, be happy and enjoy a pain free life. That's no more than common sense.

Compared with, say, seventy years ago it must be said that, as a whole, people in the West must be much healthier – we are after all, on average, likely to live about fifty per cent longer than people used to live. And, although there are penalties associated with living into old age, the streets are not crowded with aged demonstrators demanding to be 'put down'. Because of the advances in medicine we are in a much better position to control pain and fight illness.

Yet, for many people, life is still beset with a whole range of 'every-day' pains and sometimes medicine seems very hard pressed to do anything about them. I'm referring to things like backache, headache, writer's cramp (an early form of repetitive strain injury), and a vast range of aches and pains that come and go with no seeming cause and, when you are suffering from one of them, no seeming cure. Sometimes we seem to be attacked by a whole barrage of ailments that come to us without our having any control over the situation and we think of ourselves as victims. We tend to think about these sorts of mishaps as if they were the same as our being 'invaded' by bacteria and viruses. The job gives

> *For many people, life is still beset with a whole range of 'everyday' pains and sometimes medicine seems very hard pressed to do anything about them*

us backache, our partner or the children give us a headache, it's the computer mouse that gives us repetitive strain injury, and so on. What rarely seems to occur to us is that anything that goes wrong in our lives could be caused by us, by what we do, how we live. When we are suffering from these apparently random physical events, we are not happy – even if we put on a brave and cheerful face.

There are many other ways in which we can become unhappy. We may have had a difficult, even horrendous, childhood that continually blights our life. We may be failures in most, or all, that we attempt, not able to achieve much, or any, of the potential we have; we feel cheated, disillusioned, frustrated. We may fail in relationships, especially the most important ones: with parents, partners, children, the boss. We experience life as being too demanding, we can't cope, 'life' is giving us stress – not to mention grief. The list can go on and on.

Most people would think of this last list as being more 'mental' in nature and not to be treated in the same way as the physical complaints we were talking about before. Although many people will take pills of one sort or another to try and help them cope, most of us know that this will relieve the symptoms, not effect a cure. Thus, people look in another direction for help. Often this will be some form of 'talking therapy' based on one theory or another.

Over a hundred years ago F. M. Alexander began to point out the folly of dealing with the problems of life from the point of view of relief of symptoms (physical or mental), or indeed in thinking that we could divide problems into 'physical' and 'mental'.

He said that leaving accidents and invasion by germs to one side, almost all of the things we suffer from in this life are self-inflicted. It does not matter whether it is through the way we do things, meaning the way we use our physical machinery – our bodies – to get life's work done, or in the way we react to the world and our own thoughts. In both cases, we quite literally pull ourselves out of shape. It is this pulling out of shape that causes physical discomfort and prevents us from responding in a more adequate way to the world. It does not matter if the demand is a 'physical' activity (like chopping wood) or some mental response to a situation. The same *whole* self is involved.

While we are in this world, we have to exist physically and our body has to be in some 'shape' or other. The closer to the best shape for the job that we can get, the more easily we can maintain that posture during the activity (and then assume the best posture for the next activity), the less we are going to hurt ourselves and the less we are going to suffer from aches and pains or fatigue. We can learn to use our physical selves in such a way that we do not pull ourselves out of shape. No matter what the activity we can learn to get 'straight' to it. For, if we are 'out of shape' to it, we are not going to get the result we should and may very well get a result that we don't want. So, this book is all about learning not to pull yourself out of shape in your daily activities, no matter what they are.

> We can learn to use our physical selves in such a way that we do not pull ourselves out of shape

How can a book help you? Surely you have to go to an Alexander teacher to learn the Alexander Technique? Well, if that's the case, then more than ninety per cent of the population are going to be denied access to Alexander's principles. And that's a great shame. To give lessons to everyone in, say, the United Kingdom, would require the existence of hundreds of thousands of Alexander teachers – and there are less than ten thousand worldwide. Even if the right number of teachers existed, Alexander lessons are not free and the majority of people cannot afford them. And what about those who want to do things for themselves? It's worth remembering that Alexander did not have a teacher. He made just two rules for 'teaching oneself' what he had learned: 1) you must follow the same method as he did, and 2) you must give it the time that it takes. With a sound method, all it takes is time.

However, there are difficulties in teaching yourself the Alexander Technique from a book, in particular the fact that most books written about the Technique just do not have sufficient detailed instruction in them. This includes those written by Alexander, those that claim you could 'teach yourself' and those that imply that they are some sort of handbook. (They also, invariably, recommend that you go to a teacher.) This book has the necessary detail.

Another difficulty to contend with is that you are, as you will discover, pulling yourself out of shape and that you do this as a matter of *habit*. That means that you don't know of another way of doing things. It also means that you can't be given a set of exercises, say, because you will do them with the same sort of use of your body that you do other things. That is, you will pull yourself out of shape to do them. The way you normally do things 'feels'* right simply through ease of habit. So, even if you could get round the habitual way and do something in a new way, it would not feel right and you would be unlikely to continue.

This is the problem Alexander teachers spend their time helping people to overcome. A teacher may give a pupil help in a variety of ways, but the principle aim is to help people realise that they are dominated by habits of use, which feel right but are not. This is achieved, first of all, by the teacher using the hands to bring about an improvement in the way the machinery – the body – is used to keep the pupil upright. All else follows from this. It is against the background of the new experience, which the teacher is able to demonstrate is right, that previous use is thrown into relief and can be seen to be wrong. Eventually the improved use becomes permanent. The teacher has 'straightened the pupil out', as far as circumstances permit. Obviously this helps. This book, however, will show you another, teacher-less, way.

> The Alexander Technique is about the way that you use yourself in your everyday activities

The Alexander Technique is about the way that you use yourself

---

* Our subjective experience of our physical actions is mediated through very complex activities in the nervous system. By using the word 'feel' I do not mean to imply that we have some simple sense which lets us know what 'feels right' or 'feels wrong'. It is merely our colloquial way of talking about such things.

in your everyday activities. Only you can apply the Alexander Technique to yourself.

Whether you have Alexander lessons or not, you have to learn the Alexander Technique and use it in life. You can't learn to use it in the classroom, but only through applying it in real life situations. What you are taught in the classroom is how to go about the business of applying it. This book will show you that you can do that in other ways too. Be clear, though, that you can't master the Alexander Technique by memorising the words in a book. That would be like thinking you could play the violin because you'd read a book on it, even though you had never tried pushing and pulling the bow across the strings.

> The Alexander Technique is practical application or it is nothing.

This book is primarily directed at the millions of people who aren't going to have Alexander lessons. I am not, however, trying to dissuade people from having lessons in the Alexander Technique. After all, teaching people the Technique is how I earn my living. So, if you know of an Alexander Teacher and you have the money to spare and you feel so inclined, go. This book will still be very useful to you, as you will discover.

The real prize to be gained through applying the Technique to the 'problem' of living your life, is that you will cease to be dominated by habit. You will be able to direct your activities and constantly adjust your physical response so that your life and its future will truly be in your hands.

How to use this book

I f you are like me, when you get hold of a book that promises to teach you something practical you want to get straight to it. This is usually a mistake. It is always better to read the instructions before you start but I will keep this section as brief as possible.

◆You are not going to bring about astounding changes overnight and working through the book is going to take time. However, it will add just one thing to the number of things that you already have to do during the day; what we are concerned with is *how* you do the things you are doing.

Take the short route through the book the first time. Assuming that you have read 'What This Book is About', read 'How to Use This Book' to the end. (If you haven't read the previous section, read it after you have finished this one.) Next, read the summary of 'So What's the Problem?'. Then go on to read the summary of 'Lying Down' and do what it says.

Congratulations, you've started ...

When you work your way through 'So What's the Problem?', it is very important that you do understand what the problem is because the more you do, the more you will understand why the solution in this book is the right one. The more, then, you will want to apply it. However, it is not a matter of reading and learning it as if you were going to take an examination. The problem is how you do the things you do and the attitudes that you have as you do them. These things can only be appreciated and changed as you do them. The words are telling you what to look out for; come back to them time and time again. The more experience you gain of how you use yourself by working with the 'Practical Procedures', the more the words on the page will mean to

> *The words are telling you what to look out for; come back to them time and time again*

you. The more the words mean to you, the more informed your work with the Practical Procedures will be. It may be that you would like to read the whole chapter from end to end first of all to get an overview, but after that take it a few lines at a time. The object is to understand the ideas in their practical application. When you can do that, you won't need to remember the words on the page.

The longest chapter in this book is on lying down. Lying down is the most important thing for you to learn to do. It is lying down that will bring about the change of body shape. This will provide the background against which you will be able to recognise that you do things habitually and identify the way you do them. In other words, how you pull yourself out of shape all of the time, even in making the simplest movements. Only when you know this will you be able to stop doing it.

> If you can stop pulling yourself out of shape, you will be in the shape that you should be.

Lying down is the way we solve the conundrum: 'if I pull myself out of shape every time I use my machinery to do anything, how can I ever do anything to put it right?' You can't. You don't need to do anything. You do need to learn how to stop doing the things that do pull you out of shape. This achieved, you can then learn how to do the things you want to do, whatever they are, in a way that doesn't pull you out of shape.

> Lying down is the key to this. The straighter you can become, the more you will understand how it is your habit to pull yourself out of shape in everything you do.

The detail explained in 'Lying down' (p.53) is necessary. Paying very careful attention to the detail is the way we make sure that we get things right in everything we do. But you can't expect to master the detail in one fell swoop. Work on it one section at a time, until you have mastered that section, then move on. Tackle another section and add it to what you have already got. You will be surprised then to find, when you have mastered it all, that it takes about two minutes, maximum, to go through it completely without making any mistakes at all. But it isn't going to take two minutes to learn how to go through it.

As you read 'Lying down', you will find discussion of topics that will be very useful in all areas of your life.

Do you often find yourself 'drifting off', your 'mind wandering' (attention deficiency, if you like)? Lying down provides the ideal opportunity to work on this. Improvement under these circumstances will enable you to tackle the problem in other areas of life.

Most people can lie down without any trouble and will be able to follow the main procedure. But because it is such an important thing to be able to do, I want as many people as possible to do it. Therefore, I have anticipated some of the problems people may have and have included variations that may help. If you have no trouble in following the main procedure, you don't need to spend time reading the variations.

If you cannot do the lying down in any way, or belong to the group of people I suggest shouldn't do it, then go on to 'Sitting in an upright chair' for your first practical. Apply the general material in 'Lying down'.

If you don't lie down, you won't have to get up and so you can ignore the second practical.

In the lying down section I hope to establish the necessity of looking very closely at the way we do things and this approach needs to be applied to all the other practical procedures. It can be tedious to keep on repeating the same details over and over again but *you must*.

Once you have got lying down under way, start on the other practical procedures, but don't start them all at once. Tackle them one at a time. When you begin to understand the one you are working on, you can start to add another. The only time scale is the one you invent. If you try to do everything at once you will get bogged down and disheartened. You will notice that some of the other procedures are part and parcel of the lying down procedure. Bring the results of your work on them individually into that procedure and, indeed, into everything that you do.

In a short book like this, it would obviously be impossible to include every variety of human movement. Rather than give a huge list and say nothing much about each item on the list, I have restricted myself to a few basic activities and said as much as is necessary to make it possible to follow them.

When you begin to gain some confidence in doing the procedures, you will want to apply them in your everyday life. This means that you will have to do them in front of other people. For many people this becomes some sort of trial. 'What will other people think of me? Especially people I know? They will see that I'm doing things in a different way and will comment on it and maybe even laugh at me.' As for people who don't know you, they will have no idea of how you look when you are going about your everyday business. If you are straighter than you used to be, they won't know it.

As for people you know, it would be very rare for someone to say, 'Oh, you look straighter, you're just showing off.' The usual response is, 'Oh, you're looking good,' or, 'You're straighter, you look better for it'. In other words, people are usually pleased for you. When it comes to doing things in a different way you must learn that your new way of, say, taking a step or lifting something, will *feel* more remarkably different than it will actually *look*. This is because you will have paid it such a lot of attention. The more you do it, the quicker the feeling of self-consciousness will pass.

When you have reached this stage, you will know that the procedures you have gone through are right. That they work. That your use of your body and your well-being have improved. Even if you do meet someone with a negative attitude, you are not going to abandon what you are doing, and your improvement, because of it. It requires only a small act of courage to ignore negative responses. Like muscles, courage gets stronger by being exercised. You are not going through these procedures to please other people, you are going through them to improve your life. In the end, you will know what is good for you and they won't. Give them a copy of the book, then you will have done something for them.

This may seem a silly thing to say but don't keep elaborate notes. When you are giving things your conscious attention everything is being recorded in your brain. You *will* remember things and, in doing so, learn that attention is the key to memory. I have found that people who start keeping progress charts and giving themselves stars for performance, and so on, get hooked on keeping records and skimp the work. Sometimes the burden of keeping the records makes them abandon the Technique all together.

You will, of course, want to know how you are doing. First, be clear that you need to work at it regularly. This doesn't mean never having a day off, but it does mean not having very many days off. After a while, you won't want to have days off, it will be too important to you to keep things going. There is one golden rule to remember. You will not be able to feel or see very much difference day by day. Work at the practical procedures for three months, then look back and see how things have changed. Has your approach to life changed? Are you more in control? Are you having more success with the things you do? Do you find it easier dealing with people? These are the sorts of areas in which you will be able to see improvement and can count as successes. If you started with aches and pains that have now gone away, great. It's interesting, though, that once the pain is gone it is very easy for us to forget that we ever had it. And just as quickly, if we are not careful, forget *how* we got rid of it. Even if in the beginning, you started working on yourself in order to get rid of a painful condition, which has now gone, look back to see what else has changed. It will encourage you to continue for a different reason. Experience teaches that people's use of their bodies tends to get worse as time passes. If you look back and see that you do not seem to have made much progress, but see that you haven't become worse, *you are improving*. You must also, always, bear in mind

> *If you look back and see that you do not seem to have made much progress, but see that you haven't become worse, you are improving*

that improvement is a very personal thing. Never compare your rate of improvement with someone else's. It all depends on what each individual's difficulties were in the beginning. Preventing the deterioration of a condition may represent greater progress than a seemingly dramatic change for the better. For some people, change comes all of a sudden, after a lengthy period of no apparent progress, for others change comes more slowly and gradually. Keep at it no matter what – you are changing your approach to life and in the end that is what will bring long-term results.

As with all things that have general instructions, which need to be followed for success, keep on coming back to the principles outlined above.

So what's the problem?

WHAT THE PROBLEM IS 1

Almost from the beginning of our lives, we use 'tools' to deal with the world. Knives, forks and spoons, crayons, pencils and pens, pedal-cars, scooters, bicycles are all tools. To a certain extent, the number of tools we use from day to day increases throughout life. It is also clear that we need to learn how to use these things and, should there be any doubt about that, we only have to try out a new tool to discover it is true, whatever we may have thought five minutes before we started. Mastering even simple computer skills springs readily to mind, or getting the hang of a new all-in-one TV/video remote control.

What is not quite so clear is that our own bodily 'machinery' is a tool. The body is a unified collection of jointed rods (bones) moved one on the other by living 'servo-motors' (muscles). When the 'spark', the instruction, is sent from the brain down the nerves to the muscles, they twitch into action to move the bones so that we take a step, lift a fork, pedal the bicycle. What is even less clear is that we have to *learn* to use our 'machinery' effectively. Again, trying out a new activity soon shows us that this is true – everybody remembers having to learn to ride a bike! It is easy to see this in what we might call 'advanced' activities – swimming, hurdling, climbing, ballroom dancing – but the basic activities – standing, walking, running – we want to take for granted. We want to believe that somehow these activities are a given and that we get them right automatically.

> Look around you. Can you see hunched shoulders, raised chests, collapsed lower backs, unevenly distributed body weight? We don't stand straight, we don't sit straight.

In fact, 'getting straight' is about the last thing in the world that would seem possible for most people. As it is for others, so it is for most of us – look in a mirror, better still, get a trusted friend to look at you and tell you the truth.

TOO MUCH EFFORT ...

How is it that what we assume to be automatically correct, something we get right without having to try, goes so dreadfully wrong? The short answer is that we have *learned* to do these things wrongly.

> Yes, we have the capacity to stand, to sit, to walk, to run, but *how* we use our machinery to do these things is learned and it is very easy to get it wrong.

For most of us, nearly all of our waking activities depend on the ability to remain upright. Just being upright is our most basic activity. If we get this wrong, then this influences all other activities for the worse. Getting upright is not as easy as it seems. First, the bones of the legs are not bound together so that they are rigid. They are flexible. If we are to walk and climb and run, they need to be.

The only muscles in the legs that need to work to keep us upright are those in the calf and another muscle that most people have never heard of. This 'other' muscle starts from the front of the bones of the lower back. It joins onto another muscle, which comes from the inside of the pelvis. It comes out over the top of the front of the pelvis and fixes on at the top of the upper leg bone, round the back. (It doesn't have a common name – iliopsoas if anyone wants to look it up.) Between them, these muscles do everything that is necessary to keep you upright. (*Getting* upright is a different story.) They do not, singly or together, lock the knee, fix the ankle, or fix the hip. Yet all around us there are people, maybe even you, who, when standing upright, constantly lock the knee, pull themselves forward over their ankles and fix them, and then try to fix the hip joint by clenching the muscles of the bottom. What is more, they do this all quite unconsciously. It is what they have learned to do to stand up. They do this in addition to the things that it is really necessary to do.

> Standing upright is meant to be far more of a balancing act than we allow it to be.

Does it matter if we contract muscles that don't need to be working? Yes, it does, it matters a lot.

- The bony structure of the body (the skeleton) is very flexible at the joints.
- To stand upright, we need to make a certain amount of muscular effort.
- If more muscles contract than are necessary to do the job, the body's framework gets distorted.

WHAT HAPPENS IF YOU LOCK YOUR KNEES

Locking the knees and pulling forward over the ankles are distortions of the framework. The knees are pulled inward and the upper leg bones rotate inward. The weight of the body is pulled onto the inside of the feet, giving the appearance of 'flat feet' and the feet tend towards the 'toes turned out' position.

And it doesn't stop in the legs. Stiffen the legs in such a way and you will pull the pelvis round, forward and down. This pulls the lower back forward and down, thus undermining the support for the 'guts'. In compensation for the above, there will be a tendency to raise the chest. The resulting effect will tilt the upper half of the body backwards, so that you are looking out higher than the horizon and the neck is pulled forward and down to adjust the plane of the face so that you can look forwards.

None of this is good for you. In fact, it may be the basis for all sorts of discomforts and everyday ailments – headache, back-ache, neck-ache, bellyache and so on. You don't notice that you are doing it because you have been doing it for so long that you've got used to it.

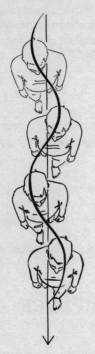

If we knew we were doing all this we could, when we came to move, 'unlock' it all. But we don't. When you start to walk, how do you shift the weight from the foot you want to move? Do you, as you should, lift the thigh up towards the upper body to take the foot off the floor and then place the foot forward and let your weight go onto it – that is, to move yourself forward? Or do you lurch to the other side first to take the weight of the foot you want to move and the leg above it and then, having put the foot down, move in a diagonal to get the weight onto it – proceeding forwards but transferring the weight in a zigzag line? The latter is far more common.

WHY DO WE GET IT SO WRONG?

When it comes to using our own machinery, not only do we not get it right, often we get it very wrong indeed. How can this be?

As we have already noted, the human frame is very flexible and remaining upright is a balancing act. We have the capacity to learn to stand upright, but to do so we have to exert ourselves through contracting our muscles. When we learn any skill, it is common-place that in the beginning either we do too little or we do too much. Too little and we don't achieve our end. Too much and — well, a variety of things can happen.

Consider throwing a stone at a target.

- Too little effort and the stone doesn't reach it.
- Too much effort and the stone overshoots. (Yes, I know that trajectory matters but let's just consider force, for the time being.)
- You judge whether you got it right or not by the effect of your shot.
- If you hit the target, that validates your effort. (Even if it was luck!)

Bowling a cricket ball is slightly more sophisticated than throwing a stone. Have you ever noticed how infrequently professional bowlers (that is to say, those who practise lots and play cricket for their living) bowl the ball at the right length and on target? If bowlers do well, we say they are 'on form'. If they don't, they are 'off form'. Comments are made about the bowler not being able to 'find his rhythm' or 'get his run-up right'. Surely if there were some infallible internal mechanism by which one could judge exactly the right degree of effort required, and the direction in which the effort should be applied, a bowler would always be on target and the ball would always be on the right length?

It doesn't happen because there is no infallible mechanism.

Consider this as an example of doing more than is necessary to achieve an end.

Writing with a pen or pencil is an activity that requires almost no physical effort. Letters at least one inch high can be formed without involving movement of any body parts other than the thumb and forefinger. Is that how you write? With almost no effort, using only the thumb and forefinger to form letters, which for most people would be large at a quarter of an inch? Or do you grip the instrument fiercely as if it would wrench itself from your fingers and run away if you didn't? Do you use the fingers to form the letters? Or do you write with the hand forming a fist and involving in its movement the forearm, upper arm and maybe even the shoulder? Do you ever get a sore finger where the pen or pencil presses? If you have to write a lot, and have done for a long time, have you a callous on the finger, often the second finger, or a permanent depression because of the pressure you exert in your grip? If you get 'writer's cramp', or a sore shoulder, or a headache when you write, does it ever occur to you that it might be because you use far more effort than is required to do the writing? Or do you look on it as a necessary evil, a consequence that is justified by the end product?

> *The essence of skill is to do as little as is necessary to gain the desired result*

You see, we judge the success of our amount of effort by whether we achieve our end or not. We do not consider whether we might have done a bit less. Yet, the essence of skill is to do as little as is necessary to gain the desired result.

To go back to the cricketing metaphor. If the batsman misses the ball, it is sufficient for the ball to strike the stumps only as hard as is necessary to make the bails fall off. The stumps being torn out of the ground and flying through the air does not make the batsman any more 'out' than if the bails had toppled gently to the ground. It is the wicket being hit and the bails falling off that makes the batsman 'out'.

Say you were writing an examination paper, how would getting writer's cramp add to the rightness of your answers? It is what you write that makes the answer correct or incorrect. Writing a good answer with less physical effort will not make it less good. A wrong answer cannot be made right because it was written with more physical effort than necessary.

If you don't understand either of these examples, consider this. In either situation, if the bowler grits his teeth as he bowls or the writer grits her teeth as she writes, what possible effect can this unnecessary effort have on the end result? It is superfluous to the end achieved, but not without consequence for the framework of the body because its effect will be to distort and indeed hinder the more necessary activity.

We have already talked about the familiar consequences of putting too much effort into writing. If you want evidence of the result of too much effort amongst sportswomen and men, just consider the number of reports of self-inflicted damage there are: 'torn' muscles, damaged tendons and ligaments, stress fractures and so on. These things happen because there is no automatic, infallible way of knowing that we are doing our activities with too much effort.

How is it that some people are very good at physical activities?

Although there are minor physical differences between us, we are all very much 'out of the same mould'. Structurally there is not a lot to choose between us. Of course, some people are tall and some are short, and some people put on weight more readily than others. Functionally, though, we are very similar. We all have a similar number and type of bones, sets of muscles attached to bones, similar nervous systems connecting to similarly structured brains. It may be true that people with a slower heartbeat make better long distance runners and powerfully built people may make better sprinters. There isn't any obvious reason, though, why one person should have better basic control of the under-lying structural mechanisms than another. It is upon this basic control of function that the more demanding skills are built.

We may be born with a predisposition to a certain 'body type', but how we use the machinery of that body is something we have to learn. If perfect use was automatically available to all of us, there is no good reason why most of us should make such an average job of physical activity at best and others worse than that.

You may wish to subscribe to some notion that what suits nature best is for there to be a minority physical élite. However, success in our long evolutionary journey has come about because we have been able to meet the tremendous challenges that an ever-changing environment has posed. Of course, it is our large brain that gives us the ability to work out our responses but it is our physical fitness that has given us the ability to implement our ideas and lies at the root of our survival. We would never have made it otherwise. It is only very recently that many of us in Western society have been able to discount physical fitness as a necessity for being able to earn our daily bread – too short a time for the ability to attain fitness to be eliminated by evolution. Don't think too narrowly about fitness. Evolutionarily speaking, it is the sort of fitness that enables a man to work at a coalface for forty or fifty years and his wife to harvest potatoes by hand; to rise at 4.30 in the morning and keep going all the time that daylight allows and then to feed and care for the children; to be able to survive for sixty years on a mediocre and scant diet with little rest and aid a new generation to continue the struggle – this is evolutionary fitness. The ability to run fast round a track, run a marathon or do 'physical jerks' is not any sort of measure of the ability to survive in a harsh world. No, for the survival of mankind as a whole, it makes more sense that the majority of us have the potential to achieve a high level of physical excellence. The conclusion we must reach is that the reason that the majority of us don't is a phenomenon of chance and an accident of learning. It is nothing to do with the smile of inborn evolutionary 'fitness' or scowl of evolutionary 'unfitness'. We are not blighted from conception to be more or less physically inept. At birth, we have as much chance as the next person to be skilled in all our physical activities.

The short answer to why some people are better at physical activities than others is that when you have a system that is very flexible and depends on balance, and the use of that system has to be learned, it is very easy to get things wrong.

The human imperative is that we must be upright – somehow. As far as survival is concerned, if that means being upright with distortion of the framework, then that will have to suffice. We are lucky that our systems compensate so well when too much effort is put into physical activity. In spite of the way we pull ourselves out of shape, we do remain upright. However, the compensating factor is more effort, which leads to rigidity and inflexibility.

In the beginning, when we are learning to stand and walk, it is probable that most of us get it right enough. Nothing can be fixed at this stage because twenty years or so of growth are still to follow. In the early years, we are constantly re-learning how to stand as our body grows and develops, altering the demand on the body. We must not, though, discount those early experiences, for what we tried once in order to satisfy the desire to stand we may well try again. It doesn't matter that we didn't think in terms of how to use ourselves, but were merely making an unconscious demand that we use ourselves to achieve some end. For instance, the baby seeing something up high that it wants will make efforts to reach it ... but not by knowing consciously that it is directing its machinery. (A moment's reflection will soon show that this is the way we still go about things in adult life.) Everything is recorded somewhere in the brain. The essence of developing a habitual response to some demand or other is that we have already done it once.

WHAT THE PROBLEM IS 2

The conceptions of the world that we are forming as we grow up have as big an effect on the way we stand and balance as our physical makeup.

There is in certain people an in-built bias towards perceiving the world as a hostile place. In other words, some of us are born with a nervous system more ready to respond to all stimuli as if they were dangerous. We say, 'Oh, he's a nervous child', or describe them as 'highly strung'. The truth is that, unless we are extremely fortunate, fear in one guise or another is a constant part of life.

It must become clear to such a child early on that practically nothing is under his or her control. People stick needles in them, parents take them off and abandon them at playgroup. When we want children to learn to swim, we immerse them in a shockingly cold sea, or swimming pools full of chlorinated water that sting their eyes. Before the children know it, they are at school being taught how to read, write and count and dance and sing, whether they will or not. All the time they are being judged and assessed on their progress. This we consider necessary if they are to survive in the modern world and we like to think that it is 'good for them'.

Most children cooperate more or less with this process, at least early on, but they do not emerge unscathed. Children get used to such things because they have no choice (after all they are compelled by law to go to school) but for many of them it is a feat of great endurance.

> To endure something means to experience the unpleasantness of it but still carry on.

For many people, the skill to endure they learned as children they retain and use through the years, living in what is to them an essentially hostile world. Modern man is bombarded day and night by stimuli (noise, responsibilities, overcrowding, poverty, unpleasant surroundings, constant flows of information), which if not threatening in themselves, can be interpreted as being so. For example, a rock concert at the proper venue may be an exciting, even awe-inspiring, experience. The same music, played by the same group, blaring from a neighbouring apartment when you do not wish to listen to it becomes a very unpleasant stimulus. Our interpretation of the stimulus determines our reaction to it.

> *If we interpret a stimulus as 'nasty' then we display a very particular bodily reaction*

If we interpret a stimulus as 'nasty' then we display a very particular bodily reaction. We stiffen the neck. This pulls the head backwards and down on top of the spine. This makes it necessary to pull the neck forward to get the face looking forward again. At the same time, we brace the legs, which turns the knees in and the toes out. Then we pull the back in (often observable as the hips being thrust forward) and raise the chest.

Familiar, isn't it? In Alexander jargon this is called 'pulling down' because the net result is that we shorten our stature. We pull ourselves down towards the floor. We exhibit the same pattern when we haven't got our balancing act right. And for the same reason. Too much muscular contraction in the system leads to pulling ourselves out of shape, out of balance, and we stiffen and fix. As an end in itself, we might make a more or less good job of learning to balance but, unless you are aware of it and know how to combat it, interpreting the world in hostile terms will always cause you to pull yourself out of shape, to pull down. You could get away unscathed if you only did it every now and then – if, when the nasty stimulus was gone, you returned to your normal, more or less balanced state – but is that how the world is? Isn't life often

> *Interpreting the world in hostile terms will always cause you to pull yourself out of shape*

one horrid stimulus followed by another, and another, and another?

Sooner or later, pulling ourselves out of shape becomes a constant factor in life and we end up responding to every stimulus as if it were unpleasant. To what degree we do it depends on how strong we think the stimulus is. Not only is this constant strain that we put on ourselves bad for our health and well-being, but by the time we reach this stage our functioning in the world is seriously impaired. We give so much attention to causing ourselves to be pulled out of shape that we have little energy left to give to the world itself, leading to attention deficit. When we cease to look outward, we become trapped in our own thoughts.

> *Pulling ourselves out of shape means that we do far more work than is necessary so that it is difficult ever to get rested enough*

Our own thoughts are the most powerful stimuli we have for pulling ourselves out of shape. Pulling ourselves out of shape means that we do far more work than is necessary so that it is difficult ever to get rested enough. We become constantly tired, chronically fatigued, as we bombard ourselves with constantly created stimuli from our own muscles and joints. Any further stimuli make us irritable and moody, so that we react badly to even well-intentioned input from others.

When nothing we do works very well we get afraid (anxious) and unhappy (depressed). For some people, the struggle of 'wrestling' one part of their body against another becomes so much of a strain that they give in. It becomes difficult to remain upright at all and they begin to slump and sag.

WHAT THE PROBLEM IS 3

It looks like all we have to do, then, is change our mind about the way we think about the world and everything will return to normal. If only it were as simple as that. There is one very powerful reason why this will not work: *habit*.

We are accustomed to thinking in terms of good habits and bad habits:

- it is good to be in the habit of cleaning your teeth morning and night
- it is good to be in the habit of cleaning your shoes at night so that you don't need to do them in the morning
- it is good to develop the habit of doing things now and not put them off until tomorrow
- it is bad to be in the habit of speaking with your mouth full
- it is bad to be in the habit of putting off until tomorrow what should and can be done today
- it is bad to be in the habit of not attending to personal hygiene

HABIT

THE WAY WE USE OURSELVES

This is not the kind of habit that we are talking about here. We are talking about the habits we have developed in the way we use ourselves in our daily activities.

When you do something for the first time, the brain is altered a little bit and preserves the pattern of the way you used your bodily machinery to do it. When you come to do that thing again, it is this retained pattern you are most likely to follow. Do something the same way twice and it is almost certain that this is the way it will be done the third time. This is the basis of *habit*.

> Habit is part of the fabric of the brain.

While we are growing children, we are constantly adjusting our use of ourselves. The rule of becoming skilled should apply: the more we understand what we are doing and the more we do it, the less effort we tend to use. This is what is sometimes thought of as practice makes perfect. But practice does not

Practice does not always make perfect

always make perfect. In fact, most people reach a ceiling of skill in any activity they undertake, which is far from what could be achieved and, often, they cannot maintain their highest level of skill consistently.

The problem is that very often when we tackle a new project, we don't know how we are supposed to use ourselves. We just assume that somehow the body will know what to do. It doesn't. What the body knows is only what we have trained it to do. So, if we learned to stand with too much effort, for instance, we will always stand with too much effort. That's what having a habit of use means. It will stop you being able to do anything in a new way.

Now you know why it is so hard to teach an old 'dog' new tricks.

THE WAY WE THINK ABOUT THINGS

If we pull ourselves out of shape because of the way we view things, we shall always pull ourselves out of shape when we are thinking about that particular thing. It doesn't matter what the subject is. It is beginning to look as if we are talking about two different systems but we are not. What we are doing is looking at the same single system but from two different points of view. The body doesn't function without direction from the 'mind' and the 'mind' cannot express itself in the world without the body. In fact even if the 'mind' and the 'body' are two different things, their activities are so inextricably interwoven that it is impossible to separate the workings of the mind and body in everyday life. The body

It is impossible to separate the workings of the mind and body in everyday life

doesn't have to *move* because the mind is working but it does have to *be*. However, the general rule is that unless we train ourselves to do otherwise, the body is constantly responding to what is going on in our mind.

There are various methods of not letting the body betray our thoughts, like having 'a stiff upper lip' to conceal the facial expression of emotion, or grasping hold of something firmly in order to not to shake with 'nerves'. These actions involve unnecessary tension and will pull you out of shape. To be rigid, as in 'keeping a straight back' to preserve courage, is just as much a way of deforming ourselves as a more obvious pulling out of shape. None of these things is desirable or necessary.

So, one way or the other, it seems that either we get the mechanics wrong or we get the thought wrong. In reality, we get both wrong at the same time. One is a reflection of the other.

We cannot know what is involved in *doing* any new activity. We can know, and need to know, that our approach to any new thing will be dominated by our past *habits*. Habits of thought and habits of use.

Let's return for a moment to the common conception of good and bad habits. It is, of course, not good (or healthy) not to wash, or prevaricate, or speak with your mouth full. And it is not bad to be prepared, clean your teeth, and do things when they can and should be done. But pulling yourself out of shape to do anything is bad for you, even if you are doing a good thing!

> *Pulling yourself out of shape to do anything is bad for you*

IMPORTANT NOTE

You may feel that you are on the horns of a dilemma. You want to do the good things in life, things you must do, but have discovered that the doing of them pulls you out of shape. *There is a solution to this problem*:

- first realise that just discovering something is bad for you does not make it worse, unless you react to the knowledge by pulling yourself more out of shape
- remember that this book has been written so that you can solve this problem
- Rome was not built in a day. There is no instant cure. You have to live with yourself as you are until you can bring about a change, and that's OK

What you do by habit comes to feel right
– even if it is wrong

In many ways, this is the most important thing about habit. Whenever we use ourselves in any activity, there is an accompanying set of 'sensations'. The word sensations is used in inverted commas because when we think of sensations we usually think of the conscious awareness of feelings such as touch, pain, smell and so on. In this case, that would be getting the wrong end of the stick.

Most of us are unaware that located in our muscles, tendons and joints there is a whole system that relays to the brain what is going on. This allows the brain to start, stop and adjust muscle contraction. Fortunately, these signals do not go directly to the conscious part of the brain. I say fortunately because if they did go to that bit of the brain we would be totally swamped by their sheer numbers. Nevertheless, it is these signals from the muscles that tell us where one part of the body is in relation to another. We don't feel it, though, even if we think we do, we just know it.

> Working together with the sensors of the inner ear and the eyes, it is this system that tells us where we are in space – not only upside down or right way up, but where we are with regard to other objects.

It is a very important sense and if we are deprived of it, as is reported to happen (fortunately very rarely), it has very dire consequences.* It is called the *proprioceptive* sense (in layman's terms, the sense of one's own physical self as a spatial object). Whenever we do anything, we take on a particular body shape and this is remembered. More importantly, it is remembered as part of

*For a personal account of someone who lost their proprioceptive sense see *Pride and a Daily Marathon*, Jonathan Cole, MIT Press, Cambridge, Mass., USA, 1995 (Duckworth, UK, 1991).

the pattern we are developing for that particular activity, its habit of use.

Getting things by habit is like taking a shortcut. The critical thing is the way we get the shortcut to work. As we start learning any activity, we give it considerable amounts of conscious attention. As we get more familiar with the task in hand and learn to do parts of it with ease, our conscious attention moves to something else. Get something sufficiently by rote and we can drift out of the 'here and now' altogether and tune into the commentary inside our head (the interior monologue). To do any 'job' (standing, walking, writing, speaking and so on), we adopt the bodily posture that we have learned. We summon this up by using our memory of what it 'felt' like to be that shape, our proprioceptive sense of that shape. This is the shortcut to the shortcut.

It doesn't 'feel' is if that is what you are doing because the activity and the 'feeling' that goes with it are like two sides of a sheet of paper. That is to say, you can't have one without the other. The activity and the 'feeling' become as one. If you like, we just get used to it.

> Another example, to give you a hint of how closely associ-
> ated action and corresponding 'feeling' are.
> The Möbius strip. A strip of paper has two sides. Give the
> strip a twist and stick the two ends together you get a
> continuous strip, which now only has one side. Try it, you'll
> see that it's true.

If you follow the procedures set out in this book, you will discover that this is true. So, because we judge our activities by whether they seem to produce the desired result (even if it is only approximately right), we think the feeling that goes with it must be right as well. This will be in spite of the fact that we may be suffering from joint-ache or backache when we do the activity. It is rare for people to make the required intuitive leap and realise that their aches and pains come because of the way that they are using themselves. We prefer to put it down to a 'weak' back (leg, foot, hip), 'my mother had the same trouble, it's in the family', or the job, or *anno domini*.

Ideally, our proprioceptive sense ought to tell us that we are getting it wrong. If our way of doing it is habitual, if the action and the feeling are one, we will feel we are right in the way we are doing it. Moreover, it will be a feeling we are used to and what is constant we tend to ignore. But even when we do something and it feels awkward we don't say, 'I must be using my machinery wrongly.' We think that there must be something in the way that we, personally, are built, that prevents us from doing it easily. If we find it too difficult, we just give up.

Ironically, this is the right thing to do, because if you persist in doing it badly, you are really going to hurt yourself and the results could be catastrophic. Sometimes people do persist, it does cause pain and ultimately they are prevented from pursuing their trade or profession.

There are a (fairly small) number of people who do have inbuilt or imposed (e.g. by trauma) defects that alter their shape away from the usual, however, the majority of people hurt themselves by the way they use themselves.

Use your bodily machinery in the right way and you will live free from the pain that using yourself badly inflicts.*

You may ask, 'If habit is a shortcut surely that's good?' Well, it would be fine if we developed habits that always involved good use of our machinery. That's quite rare.

There is a range of quality of use from perfect to absolutely dreadful. Most of us will be in the middle, somewhere between, on a good day, 'not too bad' and, on a bad day, 'awful'. In reality, somewhere between taking a pleasant stroll in the park and 'doing your back in'. (For back also read knee, elbow, shoulder, neck, wrist …)

What is it that makes the difference? First there is the state we

---

*It is unfortunately the case that occasionally the damage done through misuse, either because of the severity or the duration of it, is more than the body can restore by itself.

are in when we get out of bed. Then there are the physical demands of the day and then there is our state of mind, the way we perceive the world.

We pull ourselves out of shape (pull down) just to be upright. That is how we have learned to do it. Thus, even if we are just standing up or sitting down all day long, we are pulling ourselves out of shape just to do that. Ask yourself: How much being upright do I have to do today? How much rest is to be had? Especially important is how much 'just standing' is there to do? How long standing in the bus queue, or at the supermarket check-out, or outside the school, or at the workbench for instance?

MORE PHYSICAL ACTIVITY MAKES US PULL DOWN MORE

If our response to gravity – i.e. being upright – is to pull ourselves out of shape then to do any activity that requires more of us than just being upright will cause us to pull down more. So, how much lifting and carrying has to be done? Will it be a 'big shop'? Will you have to carry Johnny (and still push the buggy)? Will your job require more lifting and carrying than usual today? How much bending over will you do? Over the desk, over the vacuum cleaner, over the wheelbarrow, over the sink … How much twisting and turning will you do? Reversing the car, looking round the super-market, looking back for the children … There is a very simple equation. If everything you do is done with poor use, as it almost certainly is, then the harder you work the more you will pull your-self out of shape.

WHEN WE THINK THAT SOME-THING IS UNPLEASANT, WE PULL OURSELVES OUT OF SHAPE

Even if we are just standing 'thinking', if we interpret our thoughts as 'noxious', or perceive that our senses are bringing information we interpret as 'noxious', then our response is to pull down. That is, to pull down more than we would just to remain upright. The feeling, for instance, of the 'weight of the world' on our shoulders is produced by our pulling ourselves out of shape (pulling down) because of our negative responses to the world or our own thoughts. Our brain is working twenty-four hours a day interpreting the world: have you woken up to yesterday's unsolved problems? Late? With a clear head? Dozy? What sort of a day have you got to look forward to? The 'daily grind', empty, a day off, 'trouble at t'mill', another pleasant day with colleagues, looking after the children, still at loggerheads with partner, a trip to the dentist …

Now you are up, what happens? The ticket clerk is rude to you. You are carved up by a lunatic. Someone talks continuous drivel in the carriage all the way to work. The bus/train/car breaks down. You are harassed by a large white van. The children bicker all the way to school. Doom and gloom in the newspapers/on the radio/on the telly … Does the boss tear a strip off you? Does the computer go down? Do you get home with enough energy to: do the children's tea, the ironing, the washing, go for a run, have a row with partner, go clubbing, go down to the gym, flop in front of the telly, experience boredom, go to the pub, do nothing, entertain guests, fall asleep under the newspaper, spend a pleasant evening with friends in a four-star restaurant, get ready for tomorrow …

Since we react to unpleasant stimuli by pulling ourselves out of shape, the more you perceive the world to be unpleasant, the more you will pull yourself out of shape. (Note: No one is denying that the majority of examples given are, in fact, what would be considered as unpleasant stimuli. However, what we are concerned with is our perception of them as unpleasant and our consequent reaction to them.)

Remember, it is not just the fact that you work hard that is tiring, it is the way you use your machinery to do the work. And it is not just the fact that you are bombarded with

> *The more you perceive the world to be unpleasant, the more you will pull yourself out of shape*

unpleasant stimuli either from the outside world or from your own brain and body that tires you, it is the way you react to them physically. Putting the two together gives us a very 'concrete' definition of stress.

> Stress is pulling ourselves out of shape in reaction to ourselves and to the world.

Use yourself well and everything you do will make you stronger.

> **REMINDER**
> Pulling yourself out of shape through physical activity and pulling yourself out of shape through mental reaction are not different things, they are different aspects of the same thing. In everyday life, the mind and the body function as a fully integrated whole.

When we get to the end of the day, we are tired, but how tired depends on how much we have pulled ourselves out of shape. How quickly we recover depends on getting rest and freeing our mind of the troubles of the day.

Use yourself well and everything you do will make you stronger

You will though, even then, return to your base level of pulling yourself out of shape, your 'ticking over' level of pulling yourself out of shape. If you have the basic mechanics of using the machinery wrong, you will be stuck with it until you learn how to do things with good use. If you have a worrier's attitude to life, or are, as a rule, despondent, or are constantly agitated (and many other attitudes), you will still be reacting to this even though you are relaxing at home in good company.

> - It is all a matter of degree ...
> - Great demand equals great degree of pulling out of shape.
> - Less demand equals less pulling out of shape.

What you can't have is no pulling out of shape except in dreaming sleep or unless you train yourself not to do it.

NOW FOR THE GOOD NEWS ...

You pull yourself out of shape because you have learned to. Because you learned this, you can learn how to stop doing it, learn how to live your life without doing it ... That's what this book is about.

The Practicals

PRACTICAL PROCEDURES

INTRODUCTION

When using this section, always remember that the mind and body work as a single unit. There can be no doubt that the body affects the mind, after all it is the mind's means of contact with the outside world. The body is an information highway for the mind. The whereabouts of the body in space, and the relationship of one part to another, is sensed by the proprioceptive system and adds to the overall sense we have of the world and ourselves at any moment. Most of the time, we are unaware of this process.

It used to be thought, say a hundred years ago, that somehow the outside world appeared before our mind as a clear and true picture of external reality. We now know that this is not true. Because we are able to deal only with a limited amount of incoming information at any given time, there are systems within the nervous system itself for screening out signals before they get to the brain. Often it is constant 'signals' that are ignored, those that are always there like background wallpaper.

So, not only is our incoming information interpreted by the brain, it is also restricted by the system.

There are two aspects to this: 1) information, which we could receive, being blocked out, like a 'parental block' on internet information and 2) information that we cannot receive, or cannot interpret even if we could receive it. For example, we are bombarded with ultra violet light but we cannot 'see' it without special equipment, although bees can, because they have the right equipment. A satellite dish may point at the right satellite and receive the signals but, in many cases, if the 'card' isn't in the receiver, you won't get the picture you want on TV.

> We 'see' the world through the 'spectacles' of what we think we already know to be true

Everything that comes to us from the outside world and from the body is interpreted in the light of what is already stored in the mind. That is, we 'see' the world through the 'spectacles' of what we think we already know to be true. If we think about it for a bit, we know there are all sorts of pieces of information that we've picked up along the way and accept as true, which may not be. We have probably never bothered to find out whether they were true or not. However, that does not stop us acting on them as if they were true. A very trivial example …

Most of us enjoy 'spoonerisms' and sometimes we may use them to amuse our children. We may go past a field and say, 'Look at the runny babbits.' Usually the children will protest that we've got it wrong and it becomes a family joke. I once knew a well-educated person who regularly used to say: 'I looked into every crook and nanny.' One day it dawned on me that this was not the usual family joke, but that the person really did believe this was the correct expression. I asked and found it was so: 'Dad used to say it when we were children. It never occurred to me that he was pulling our legs.'

What matters is that you understand that your view of the world is not a photograph of how it really is. Your view of the world has an awful lot to do with your life so far. I want to look at one special aspect of this that will cause us problems if we don't understand it.

When you begin, the main reason for following the practical procedures will be to find out what you do with your bodily machinery when you do something. Do I brace my knees? Do I hold my breath? Do I grit my teeth? Do I close my eyes? And so

> When you begin, the main reason for following the practical procedures will be to find out what you do with your bodily machinery when you do something

on. If we don't know what we do, we can't tell whether or not we do something with good use or poor use. If we do things with poor use we must know exactly what it is that makes it poor use because that is what we have to stop doing in order to change our activity to good use. The problem is that what we do, whether it is with good use or poor use, is habitual. What we do habitually, we get used to. What we get used to 'feels' right.

We are already prejudiced to believe that:

- what feels 'right' is right
- what feels 'different' is wrong
- what feels 'wrong' is wrong

In the beginning, it is not possible to tell whether a way of doing something is right or wrong by feeling alone. You must make the conscious decision, right from the start, that in the process of exploring the procedures you will suspend your judgement as to what is right or wrong as far as your use of yourself is concerned. As you go through the procedures, you will come to understand that you cannot rely on your previous experience to determine what is good use or poor use:

- what feels 'right' may be wrong
- what feels 'different' may just be unfamiliar
- what feels 'wrong' may not be wrong

But – beware, the general rule must be, if it causes *pain* it is *wrong*.

> Beware, the general rule must be, if it causes pain it is wrong

In order for us to get an idea of what we do

habitually, we must introduce new information. This will allow us to view our habitual behaviour against an unfamiliar background.

We have said that our habit is to use too much muscular contraction when we are upright, which pulls us out of shape. A sensible way to start, then, would be to have some sort of procedure to go through that would enable us to straighten ourselves out. Then we might be in with a chance of learning what it is we do that pulls us out of shape. Once we know what it is that pulls us out of shape, we should be able to learn to stop doing it. Then we would be in a position to learn what to put in its place – this often means *not doing anything*.

Remember, a lot of the time we are doing *more* than is necessary.

SPECIAL NOTE ABOUT PRACTICAL PROCEDURES

Do not be put off by the amount of space the procedure takes up on the page. It takes a lot of space to describe an activity in some detail. The activity itself may only take a few seconds to perform.

If you want to get the benefit, you must take the short time it requires to master the detail.

PRACTICAL PROCEDURE 1

LYING DOWN

> **NOTE**
> 1. Read the procedure through to the end before attempting to do any of it. It will only take a few minutes.
> 2. It may turn out that it is not possible for you to lie on the floor (for a variety of reasons). Or it may gradually become clear that it is not a good idea for you to lie on the floor. There is a variation for those who cannot lie down on the floor at the end of this procedure that should make it possible to achieve the same benefit.

INTRODUCTION

It is well known that when we get a good night's sleep we are taller the morning after it than we were when we went to bed. This may not seem a lot in itself, but it gives us a clue as to where we need to start. The most reasonable explanation of why this should be the case is that during dreaming sleep most of our muscles are as relaxed as they can be. If we sleep in a reasonable position and our bed is not in too bad a condition, the muscles let go and allow gravity to push the body against the bed and 'flatten' it out.

So, let's exploit this. We are going to lie on a firm surface to encourage flattening, but we are not going to sleep. We could get down onto the floor by falling down all of a heap, but it wouldn't do us much good. In fact, in order to minimise the constant pulling out of shape we do, we have to be very careful about how we get onto the floor.

The chief function of our muscles is to keep us upright against the force of gravity. If we lie down, they no longer have to perform this job. As soon as we lie down, the muscles working to hold us up can let go. This includes those we were using to hold ourselves up, which we didn't need to use. Although muscular activity stops at once, it takes time for the body to straighten out.

> Lying down on the floor once is not going to overcome the pulling out of shape of a lifetime. But lying down the first time starts the process.

PRELIMINARIES

Clothing

This procedure can be done with or without shoes. It is *not recommended* that you lie down in jeans, which are generally stiff and non-pliable, nor that you lie down with a belt or braces on. Both of these can dig into the back and be very uncomfortable, and braces can cause the trousers to 'ride up' when you are lying on your back. Also avoid thick belt loops at the back of skirts and trousers. If you are uncomfortable, you will pull yourself out of shape.

Lying down, however, is an activity that we want to be able to carry out during the course of our normal day, so it is not a 'special clothing' activity. Just bear the above in mind. You may get away with jeans – but you won't lie down for very long with something sticking in your back.

Where and on what?

You will need a floor space as long as you are tall and at least twice as wide as you are. Do not lie on a concrete, wooden, or tiled floor without putting a covering on it. A camping mat or a doubled blanket will serve for you to lie on, but a floor with a carpet and underlay is best.

Where you are going to lie down should be 'out of the way' so that you will not be disturbed for up to twenty minutes. This includes not being disturbed by pets. If you have no choice but to lie down in a place that is not very warm, you will need a blanket to cover you. We tend to stiffen against the cold, which is the opposite of what we are trying to achieve in lying down.

What we are trying to achieve

We are trying to be in a lying down position that will let us take the greatest advantage of gravity pressing down on us to straighten us out. However we get down onto the floor, and however we lie on the floor, the instant we get down, the muscles that have been holding us up against gravity will stop contracting. We do not, though, want to lie down any old how. We do not want to lie on our fronts, for instance (think of it as being a 'downtrodden' position: face in the mud, difficult to move, pressure on the vital organs, difficult to breathe). We do want to be straightened out front to back because we tend to shorten ourselves in front and round over at the back, when we pull ourselves out of shape. Therefore, we want to lie on our backs.

If we lie on our backs with our legs outstretched and no support under the head, several things happen. Our feet tend to fall out to the side pulling our legs round with them. The weight of the legs pulls the pelvis round and arches the lower back (pulling us out of shape). This can only be overcome by muscular activity, thus removing the advantage of lying down. The head tends to loll back. The head being back tends to arch the neck forward (again, pulling us out of shape). Note, this head back position may be correct for 'mouth to mouth resuscitation'. It is difficult, however, to believe it has any other benefits. Therefore, we want to lie on our back with our legs up and our head supported. This will give us the position we need to take greatest advantage of the situation.

The headrest
You will need some paperback books.

- These should be about the thickness of a two hundred page novel. Say about half an inch. (The content doesn't matter; it's the thickness that counts.)
- You need enough to make a pile that is as high as about the width of your own hand.
- They should be arranged so that all the spines are underneath each other.
- The books should have some 'give' when you press them between your fingers.
- Have a couple of books to spare.

You will also need a woollen scarf or piece of cloth about the same size or thickness. Fold this until it is about the width and thickness of one of the books.

Positioning the headrest

Go to where you are to lie down. Walk to where you want your head to be. Take a step to the side with one foot or the other so that there is a distance of nine to twelve inches between your heels.

Take one step backwards with one foot or the other. (The step should be big enough so that when you put the foot on the floor, the toes of the foot you are stepping back with are behind the line of the heel of the front foot.)

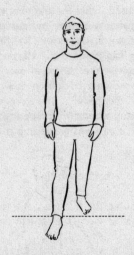

Let the weight be even on both feet. You are going to lower your height by letting both knees go at the same time:

- don't deliberately try to bend the knees, let them go
- gravity will take you down
- your muscles will act to slow you down unless you want to

drop like a stone – not recommended
- the knee of the back leg will come into contact with the floor. There will be more or less a right angle at the other knee
- the toes of the back foot will be bent forward – flick them back (if you find this difficult to do with shoes on, then either start again, having taken your shoes off, or next time you do the procedure do it without shoes)

Without bending the torso, come forward from the hips, the head going forward in an arc, and place the pile of books on the floor where your head is to be. The forward movement should come from the hips. (The hip joint is the one where the bone of your upper leg joins onto the pelvis – your 'tailor's' or 'dressmaking hips' are at the top rim of the pelvis, about four to six inches higher than the hip joints. If you bend from here, you will round over. Not what we are after.) Place the folded scarf beside the pile of books together with the spare books. The spines of the books should face away from you. (If you find it difficult to come forward from the hips when on one knee, then you should get onto both knees. This procedure is described under 'Getting onto your back' below.)

Bring your back into the upright, like the spoke of a revolving bicycle wheel.

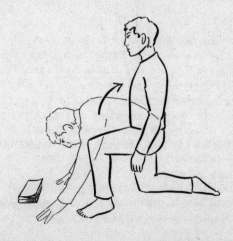

Stand up by sending your head straight up towards the ceiling. Do not tilt your head back.

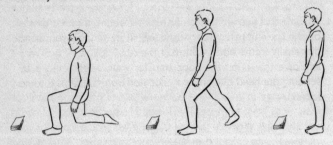

> **NOTE**
> If you find lowering your height by letting the knees go difficult, there are four variations to the procedure at the end of this section.

GETTING ON TO YOUR BACK

You should now be standing with the books at your feet.

1. Turn round.
2. Walk, in a straight line, your torso's length away from the books (about two or three steps). You will learn to judge this distance very accurately by eye. (If you really have a great deal of difficulty in judging the right length, cut a piece of string the length of your back from the top of the pelvis to the base of the skull. Lay it on the floor, stretched out, to the left or right of the books – not on the bit of floor you are going to lie on – starting from the line of the books and in the direction that you are going to walk.)
3. Turn right or turn left.
4. Take one step forward with one foot or the other. This step should be long enough for the heel of the front foot to be in front of the line of the toes of the back foot.

5. Lower yourself onto one knee as described on pp. 56–7.

Now to getting the other knee onto the floor.

1. Assume that you are facing north. If it is your right knee that is on the floor, transfer your weight onto it by sending your head diagonally to the north-east. (Let the torso follow.) If it is your left knee that is on the floor, transfer your weight onto it by sending the head diagonally to the north-west. (Let the torso follow.)

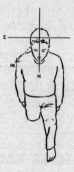

2. As the weight comes off the foot, lift the leg by sending the knee straight up to the ceiling and place the knee next to the other one.
3. Come back into the vertical by sending the torso back along the diagonal.

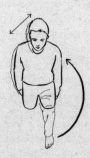

4. You should now be on both knees with the upper legs vertical and the torso vertical above that. If the legs and torso are not vertical, bring this about by sending the head up towards the ceiling and let the torso follow. Do not tilt the head back.

You are now going to sit on the floor.

1. Send your bottom diagonally backwards and down to the space to the right of your ankles. If you turned left instead of right (see above), then you will send your bottom to the left of your ankles.

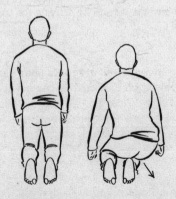

2. At the same time, put your arm out to the side so that it comes to the floor in line with your ankles and bottom, and put your hand on the floor.
3. Straighten the legs a little so that there is a right angle at the knee.

You are now going to lie on your side on the floor.
1. Bring your free hand across and put it on the floor next to your other one. This means letting the outstretched arm bend at the elbow.
2. Using both hands alternately, 'walk' yourself along with them until you are lying on your side. It is important to make sure that you are lying on your hip.
3. When you are nearly there, stretch out your right arm in front of you and rest your head on it. It will be your left arm if you turned left.
4. You should now be lying on your side with legs crooked and your head level with the books, which are a few inches away from you, behind your head.

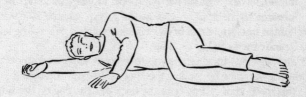

You are now going to roll over onto your back.
1. The movement, which should be continuous, must start with your head then follow through into the neck, then into the torso, then the pelvis and finally the legs – which you do not straighten. The temptation is to do it legs first. Don't. It will twist and compress the back and, if you have a bad back, the twisting will cause pain. Start from the head.

If all has gone to plan, you will be lying on your back with your head on a pile of books, your feet on the floor and your legs like an upside down 'V'.

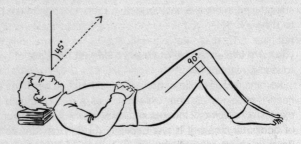

If the books aren't quite where your head is:

1. Let your head rest on the floor while you reach for the books with one (or both) of your hands.
2. Put a hand onto the top of your head so that the fingers are going down the back of the head.
3. Lift the head with the hand while thinking of the head rotating forward at the top of the backbone. Do not pull the neck forward.
4. Put the books under your head.
5. Release the head back – slowly.

If your legs did straighten as you rolled over, lift them into position one at a time by sending the knee up towards the ceiling.

This method of getting onto the back by first lying on the side should be suitable for most people including those with bad backs. This way of getting onto the floor may seem fussy, but it will get you on your back without hurting you or making the mechanical conditions you started with worse.

Adjusting the position

Ideally, you want to be able to get onto your back without having to make any but the smallest adjustments. However, it may be necessary to adjust the height of the books under the head and the position of the feet.

Adjusting the height of the books

There is a positive reason for having a pile of books under the head. It is not just to stop the head lolling back. When we are standing up, there is a best attitude, or relationship, of the head to the neck. When you are standing up, you almost certainly do not have it. There is a way of promoting it when we are upright, as you will see later, and we can use the height of the pile of books to start promoting it.

Recommending a pile of books about the same height as your hand is wide results from experience; as a rule of thumb it is reasonably accurate. However, sometimes a considerable number of books are needed. It just depends on how far forward and down you habitually pull your neck. Sometimes, not often, fewer books are needed.

Try the following diagnostic tests while you are lying down. First, as before, make sure the pile of books is straight and that the spines are pointing away from you. Second, make sure that the bulge at the back of the head (the occiput) is in the centre of the books. Where are you looking? If you are looking straight up or backwards, the books are too low. Add a book and assess again.

The nodding test

If you are now looking forward of vertical, try the nodding test.

- Do you have to pull your head round forward a long way to nod? Answer 'yes', still too low. Add a book. Test again.
- If you can nod by getting your head to go a little way back and freely forward, and then return to where you started, the pile is probably the right height.
- If you can't nod, the books are probably too high. Take a book out and test again. Don't forget where you should be looking. (There is a possibility that the books may be too far away – see below.)

Test this in turn with the following procedure.

The fist test

- Gently roll one hand into the shape of a fist and see if you can put it diagonally between your chin and the top of the chest. If

you can, the height of the books is probably OK.
- If you can with lots of room to spare, the books are too low. Add a book. Test again.
- If you definitely can't get your fist in, and the gap is, say, an inch too small, try nodding again. Is the head really going freely forward or is it tight? The books are probably too high.
- Take a book out. Test again.

The speaking test
- Try speaking (a nursery rhyme maybe – anything at all will do). What is the quality of the voice like?
- Is it free and resonant? The books are probably the right height.
- Or is it a bit tighter than usual? If it is, the books are probably too high.
- Take a book out. Test again.
- If the books are too low, it may feel awkward when you speak.
- Add a book.
- Test again.

If you are looking forward of vertical and

- you can nod freely
- you can get your fist between your chin and your chest
- and your voice doesn't sound tight, then

you have probably got a good approximation to the right height of books for you.

When you've got the height of the books right, replace the top book wth the folded scarf, otherwise it can be very hard on your head. Start with this height of books next time, including the scarf from the outset.

(If you feel that the neck is being stretched, the books are probably a tiny bit too far away. Make sure that the 'bulge' (the occiput) of the back of head is resting in the centre of the books.)

It is worth taking this trouble to get the height of the books right. If you do, you have probably got it right for several weeks or months. (Maybe, if you had, say, only two books to begin with, for ever.) Most of us, however, must expect the height to vary. The tendency over the months is for the pile to get smaller as you straighten out. It doesn't mean you are not straightening out if it doesn't, though.

In time, you may be able to lower the height of the pile by a whole book within a single lying down session. Book height is a good guide to how much you have pulled yourself out of shape since you last did the lying down procedure.

Adjusting the feet and legs

Shoes or no shoes

I said, earlier, that you can go through this procedure with or without shoes. You've also seen that letting the knees go and being on your knees with shoes can be difficult for some people. Why then not do it without shoes and be done? Firstly, this is a procedure that you want to be able to do anywhere, provided you've got the space, your books and scarf, and you're dressed appropriately. You could do it on the lawn, in the park, on a firm sandy beach (provided these places are level), in the back of a van, on the floor in the office, and so on. Away from home (e.g. in the office) taking the shoes off may be inconvenient and if you haven't learned to do the procedure with your shoes on, you may be put off.

The other reason affects every time you lie down. It depends on what you are lying on of course, but shoes do not slip as easily as the 'socked' or 'stockinged' foot. If you are going to do the lying down without shoes on then you need to make sure that there is something that your feet won't slip on where your feet are going to be. I have recently discovered that 'rubber' mesh, which is put underneath rugs to prevent them from moving, or in the boot of the car to stop things sliding about, is good for resting the feet on to prevent them slipping. (I am obliged to my student Janyce Hawliczek for this discovery.)

If your feet are too far away from your bottom when you are

lying down, there will be a tendency for them to slip away whatever is on your feet. The cure for this is not to draw your feet up closer to you and hold them there with tension. We want the legs to be free of muscular effort.

Positioning the feet
The best position of the leg requires the feet to be flat on the floor with a right angle at the knee.

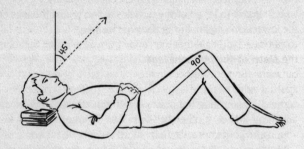

If you got that angle right when you were sitting next to your ankles, it should still have been there when you rolled over. If

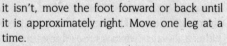

it isn't, move the foot forward or back until it is approximately right. Move one leg at a time.

You will probably have to adjust the distance between your feet. If your feet are too close together, the knees will tend to fall out and you will want to hang onto the legs. We don't want this to happen. The distance between your feet should be the same as when you are standing up: about six inches.

Adjust the distance by lifting the foot (sending the knee up to the ceiling) and putting the foot down in the right place. You are better off adjusting both feet rather than just one. Only the leg should move; the torso should remain still. The feet should have the weight of the leg evenly spread: on the heel, outside edge of the foot and across the ball of the foot. (If it isn't now, it will come in due course.) Don't push onto them or try to push them into the right place. There ought to be an angle between the feet of about forty-five degrees.

'Balancing' the legs

If you can get the position of the feet right, the legs ought to balance. We need them to balance because if they don't, we won't be able to let go of the muscles in the top of the legs or in the lower back. Again, this is not what we want. Let the legs fall in towards each other, rather than away from each other. Sometimes the state of your personal mechanics causes your legs to fall outwards. Sometimes people are in the habit of pulling the legs apart. If either of these is the case, adjust the legs so that they are vertical (by adjusting the position of the feet) and then let them fall in towards each other. Let them rest together at the knee. As your overall use improves, they will come into balance.

If you pull the legs in together, let them fall out again until they are vertical. If you can, let them balance there. If you can't, let them fall in so that they rest on each other. In time, they will come into balance.

Getting the torso right

Only move the torso if you really have to. If the torso isn't right, it is either a) because when you rolled over from being on your side, you didn't do it in the correct order (head, torso, hips, legs) and have become twisted, or b) you are feeling the shape you are. In either case try to leave it alone – don't fidget. If some piece of clothing has become rucked up, try to pull it straight without moving the torso. If you must move, do it by rolling (head first, then torso, then hips, then legs), but only do this if it is vitally necessary, if lying there is intolerable.

What you are going to feel, mostly, is the shape you are. You may note that your back is arched, or that your shoulders are uneven, or that

> *Change of shape must be passive*

the back of your shoulders are not on the floor, or only one is, and many other things no doubt. This is the situation you are trying to improve. Don't try to *do* anything about it. The change of shape must be passive.

If you *do* anything directly – force the shoulders back or the back down – you won't be able to maintain the position and it will make matters worse.

> The change of shape will come if you do the lying down procedure regularly over a long enough period.

What shall I *do* with my arms?
Let the hands rest palm down on your front, about the level of the bottom of the ribs.

VARIATIONS

To be used if you find it difficult lowering the height by letting the knees go.

Variation 1
1. Take an ordinary chair (and the books and scarf) to where you want your head to be.
2. Sit on it facing the direction that your head will be. Both feet should be flat on the floor with a right angle at the knee.
3. Make sure that there is a distance of about two feet between your heels.
4. Come forward from the hips (as described above).
5. Place the books on the floor between your feet (as above).
6. Place the scarf and spare books next to the pile of books.
7. Come back into the upright (as above).
8. Stand up by adjusting the distance between the feet to about six inches. Move one foot back a little and the other foot forward a little. Both feet should still be flat on the floor.
9. Use your hands to help you position yourself as far forward in the chair as you can without slipping off (see p. 143).

10. Send your head up above your feet to where it would be if you were standing up. Do not tilt the head back.

Note, getting out of the chair will be treated as a practical procedure later (p. 139).

11. Move the chair and go back to stand in front of the books.

Variation 2

1. Take an ordinary chair (and the books and scarf) to where you want your head to be.
2. Place the chair in front of you, just the other side of where you are going to put the books down, with its back towards you.
3. Put the books and scarf on the seat of the chair where you will be able to reach them when you are on your knees.
4. Place your hands on the top of the back of the chair.
5. Follow the procedure for lowering the height (p. 144).
6. If the chair is not quite far enough away to stop your head hitting it, move it away a little.
7. After you have put the books and scarf down, move the chair back towards you. If necessary, place your hands on the top of the back of the chair.
8. Stand up by sending the head up towards the ceiling, use the hands to steady you (and only as a last resort to get you vertical). See Variation 3 below.

If you are tempted to have the seat of the chair towards you see Variation 3.6 below.

Variation 3

1. Take an ordinary chair, or two ordinary chairs, to where you want your head to be.
2. Place one chair, with its back towards you, to your left (or right), with you standing in front of the place where you want the headrest (pile of books) to be.
3. If you are going to use two chairs, you place one to the left and the other to the right.
4. Place the books and scarf on the seat of one of the chairs where

you will be able to reach them when you are on your knees.

5. The chairs are there to make you feel secure and so that you can use your arms should the need arise.

6. Place a hand on the top of the back of the chair. (One hand on each chair if you are using two.) You may be tempted to have the seat(s) of the chair(s) facing inwards towards you. Don't give in to it. Unless you can let your knees go so that your hands come naturally into contact with the seat as you are lowering your height, the desire to shorten to put your hand on the seat before you start lowering your height will be very great. If, in spite of what I say, you are going to do this anyway, then make sure you use two chairs and put your hands on them at the same time. At least you shouldn't be leaning over to one side.

7. Follow the procedure for lowering your height, placing the books and scarf, and coming back into the upright.

8. To get back on your feet again, it is vitally important that you want your head to go up towards the ceiling as a priority. Do not tilt the head back.

9. If you need to use your arms to get up, wanting the head to go up to the ceiling will make it easier. Don't just go 'heave-ho' with the arms. It's the leg muscles that get you up.

10. Move the chairs and go back to stand in front of the books.

Variation 4
1. Get someone to put the books and scarf in place for you.
2. Stand in front of the books.

SHOULD YOU LIE DOWN?

Should you lie down? Yes, if you can. Most people really like lying down. However, some people find lying down a difficult and even unpleasant thing to do, for reasons other than the difficulties involved with getting onto the floor.

> If you are one of those for whom lying down on a firm
> surface is a problem, then give more attention to the other
> procedures.

If you are very 'bony' and find it uncomfortable on the floor, put a
thicker covering down – a duvet, or a quilt, two doubled over
blankets, or some variation. Up to a couple of inches of soft
covering will probably do the trick. When you lie down, the inner
contents of the abdomen – your 'guts' – not only fall back
towards the floor, but also in the direction of the head. This
means that movement of the diaphragm can be restricted. This is
quite important because if the diaphragm doesn't move at all you
stop breathing. When we are lying down, the amount our
diaphragm needs to move will be very small, because our demand
for air will be small, so for most people this will never ever be a
problem. But if, when you are on your back on the floor, you find
that your breathing is restricted to an uncomfortable degree (for
example, if you are pregnant), don't panic – your breathing won't
stop – but do get up. Carefully, in the method described later.

If you are pregnant, it may be the case that lying down is just
uncomfortable because of the shape you are in, nothing to do
with floor coverings and weight. Some people who have had no
trouble lying down before, do find it very uncomfortable when
they are pregnant and have to stop. For others, it isn't a problem.
In the later stages of pregnancy, though, when the baby is getting
very big, the bulge may restrict the breathing too much.

Occasionally, for no obvious reason, some older people experience interference with the breathing. Breathing comes first. Get
up carefully and, again, don't panic. (The method for getting up
will be explained shortly.)

It may be that you have difficulty getting on to the floor.

There can be many reasons for this, for example:
• for one reason or another your joints don't work as they used to
  (or should)

- even with the aid of the chairs you are too unstable (or fearful of being too unstable)
- it makes too great a demand on the muscles (or you think it will)

One solution is that you have a very firm, unyielding, orthopaedic bed. If you haven't, don't go out and get one. Sleeping on a very hard surface is an art. It is an art not worth practising unless you really have to.

HOW TO LIE DOWN ON A HARD BED

> Note, some people with bad backs may find this preferable to lying on the floor.

Place the books on the midline and at one end of the bed, about six inches from the end. (Put the scarf and the spares next to the pile.) Use your eye to see where you need to sit. (Or use the piece of string method.) Stand with your back to the bed and sit down, a little this side of the midline. Lie on your side – use your hand if necessary. Your head should be level with the books. Bring your legs up onto the bed in the crooked position. Roll over onto your back as described earlier (p. 61).

A SECONDARY REASON FOR LYING DOWN EVEN IF YOU CAN'T LIE ON A FIRM SURFACE

The main reason for lying down on a firm surface, as has already been said, is to get the 'straightening out' effect. There is a secondary reason for doing it.

- We tend to get up in the morning and then just keep going.
- We need to take rests more often than we do.
- Fatigue is not a straightforward thing and has less to do with muscles than most people think.
- The nervous system gets fagged as well. Which means that it

becomes less efficient rather than that we 'feel' anything. We simply don't function quite so well.

- Just as we relieve the demand on the muscles that hold us up by lying down, we also relieve the consequent demand on the nervous system (which triggers the necessary constant contraction of the muscles).

Muscular and nervous activity is a chemical process. Some of the chemicals involved are recycled, some turn into a waste product. A period when nothing much is going on allows the body to sort out the chemistry and get rid of waste. Therefore, even if you can't lie on a firm surface, you may find that you can lie on a bed or on a sofa because of the extra give. Sofas are often firmer than beds. Lie down for the rest in the same way as you would if you were lying on the floor. However, you will probably find books too unstable and will have to use pillows or a cushion. If the bed is too soggy, it probably isn't worth it.

Those who can lie on a firm surface may also find it worth doing when they are in circumstances where they can't lie on the floor: some hotel rooms for instance.

WHAT HAPPENS WHEN YOU FIRST LIE DOWN?

The muscles stop working immediately, but you don't straighten out at once. So the first thing to do is just lie there for a bit.

For many people, the first thing that happens is that the eyes close and you may breathe quite deeply. This is sometimes accompanied by a 'numbness' of mind. Not a blankness, more like a shut down. This lasts a very short time. There is sometimes a wooziness. Unless you are ill and wooziness is a symptom of what you've got, this will also pass quite quickly. You may even sleep, and indeed dream, for a few minutes. There may be the feeling that your limbs and body are slowly draining out, as if they had been full of water.

All these things are symptoms of tiredness and the more tired you are, the longer the symptoms will last. Sometimes this is to do with age because the older we are the more slowly we recover. If you fall deeply asleep for a long time, this is, you will not be surprised to hear, a sure sign of being tired (if you are not ill) and you would have been better off lying on a bed or sofa.

Learn to assess how tired you are. Ask yourself: am I going to lie down for 'a straighten' and a rest? Or am I so tired I must lie down for a rest first. Falling asleep for any length of time on a firm surface, on your back, with a pile of books underneath your head is not conducive to comfort. You will wake up cold, numb and with a 'stretched' feeling in the neck. All of which you may have reacted to with tension – and pulled yourself out of shape, defeating the object of the procedure. So, if you feel you could do with half an hour's sleep, lie down on your bed or the sofa.

> The longest you should lie down on the floor for is twenty minutes. Whatever straightening is going to happen will have happened by then. Very soon after this, the numbness and drop in body temperature begin.
>
> Life is not about lying on the floor. Lying on the floor is a means to an end, it is not an end in itself.

WHAT TO DO WHILE YOU ARE LYING DOWN

INTRODUCTION

When you are recovered from the initial moments of lying down, your mind will become active again. It may seem to you that your eyes have just opened and that you can 'see'. The reason for this is that your facial tension will be letting go as will tension in the muscles that move the eye.

You may also realise that you need to go to the loo. Get up and go, then lie down again, following the procedure. Most people 'hold on' instead of going as soon as they realise that they need to 'go'. This is probably a habit from child-hood. Going immediately is preferable. Holding on is just another way of pulling yourself out of shape. If you hold on you can't 'undo'. Undoing is what you are lying there for.

We must give our habitual thoughts a rest too

Remember that our body is our means of expressing to the world what is in our minds. So when your mind becomes active again, you will start thinking your habitual thoughts. With your habitual thoughts go your habitual muscular tensions. The only way to stop this is not to think the thoughts. We must give our habitual thoughts a rest too.

> When we are lying down, not thinking our habitual thoughts, and we are directing our attention, we do not need to *do* anything to relax. We *are* relaxed.

No demand equals no activity. (In truth, just enough activity to keep us ticking over physiologically.) All we need to do is get the lying down set-up right; gravity and our physiology will do the rest.

All the usual relaxation 'games': 'think of your back getting warm and going soft' or 'march the little soldiers out of the end of your toes' are merely thought distraction. They prevent us from thinking our habitual thoughts. Even then we will try and 'do' the games in our habitual way. Thought distraction games will not train us consciously to direct our thought.

STAYING IN THE 'HERE AND NOW'

What we need to learn to do is attend to being in the 'here and now'. In one way this is a silly thing to say because we can't be in any other place but the place we are in, and we can't be anywhere at all at any other time but now. Our thoughts give us the impression that we can, though.

If we are not actively directing our thoughts, we will be 'drifting off' (wool gathering, mind-wandering, day-dreaming). We consider this 'thinking'. Drifting off is always an excursion into our past and our past is completely dominated by our habits of use. When we drift off, we may not be wholly aware of where we are, and have no sense of time. Wherever we may 'feel' we are, our body is always someplace in the physical world. And, unless we train ourselves otherwise, our body is always responding to our habitual thought. When we drift off, we pull ourselves out of shape in response to the patterns of use we have established in the past.

Training ourselves to stay in the here and now

If it is our habit to drift off, it is going to take time to teach ourselves to direct our attention. Only you can teach yourself to do this.

The way the brain works

- Even in our deepest sleep the brain is active.
- In our waking life, we can be conscious or unconscious of what we are doing.
- In practical jobs needing constant problem solving, we consciously attend to what we are doing all the time.
- This is probably true with what we think of as 'mental' tasks of the same nature.
- When the brain has had enough of something for the time being, it will 'jump'. We find ourselves thinking about something else – our mind has wandered.
- The brain does not necessarily work

> *It is going to take time to teach ourselves to direct our attention*

in a straight line, however much we would like it to sometimes.

- In addition to any particular thing that we consciously want to retain in our memory, all sorts of other information gets simultaneously stored alongside it, unconsciously.

An example

As we are learning something for a history test before going to school:

- we read that William beat Harold at the Battle of Hastings in 1066 and became William the Conqueror
- we smell grilling bacon
- we are trying to put our shoes on without taking our eyes off the book (and without undoing the laces!)
- we're thinking the weather is great and it is cruel to send a child to school on such a day
- we can hear our baby brother in his cot screeching for attention
- we feel agitated because even though we don't want to go to school much, we don't want to be late either
- we're cross with Dad for taking so long in the bathroom and making us all late

We may pay not much attention to anything else but the text we are learning unless it overrides our main focus of attention and by the time we have got to school, except perhaps for an agitation 'hangover', everything else will have left our consciousness. Eventually, test over, we will forget everything about the early morning experience. Yet, in later life we will not be able to fathom why the smell of grilling bacon always reminds us that 'it was one in the eye for Harold in 1066'. It will be the smell of the bacon (or a crying baby) that brings back the memory.

Conclusion

The truth is that wherever our attention is now, where it will be in a few seconds (or less) does not just depend on where it should go logically. All information current and stored is taken into account. The complex of nerve cells, which is active at this moment, is in contact with hundreds of thousands of other nerve complexes. Which set of cells is activated next in any sequence takes all available information into account. It may be some utterly trivial detail that leads us 'astray' from 2 + 2 = 4, to 2 + 2 = the memory of a peaceful trip on the river drinking wine with friends.

How do we stop 'drifting off'?

We can take precautions against inattention by inputting lots of relevant information associated with what we are doing now, by loading the system in our favour, expecting and screening out random intrusions as they occur. Taking rests from the activity we are doing also helps, because the problem gets worse as we get fatigued (which may be quickly when we are doing something unfamiliar and/or difficult).

The dangers of familiarity and boredom

There is another reason why our attention is distracted: familiarity and boredom. If we are doing a very familiar job (whether it comes into the 'physical' or 'mental' category), which we can do 'standing on our heads', we will tend to do it with 'our eyes closed'. Eventually we get tired of doing the same thing over and over again, however complicated the job. If we are forced to pay attention to it nevertheless, it can lead to feelings of boredom. This can apply to managerial or educational (even higher educational) tasks as much as to those involving a conveyor belt or some other routine, mentally undemanding job.

Boredom setting in is probably a signal that the brain needs a change of stimulus. But the feeling of boredom itself is a stimulus that can be reacted to. It is an unpleasant stimulus and we will tend to react to it by pulling ourselves out of shape. The irritation and other symptoms, which we sometimes experience alongside boredom, are a result of the pulling out of shape. We can pull ourselves out of shape to the

> The feeling of boredom is a stimulus that can be reacted to

point of standstill and be reluctant to start a job again once we stop. We may attempt to do the job with as little input as possible and drift off frequently. This can lead to error and inefficiency, 'going slow' and outright skiving.

The ideal cure is to avoid the situation. If that isn't possible, then frequent rests and changes help. If we have, in the end, to endure boredom, then the cure is to learn not to pull ourselves out of shape under these conditions. This is not done overnight. Familiar and easily done tasks require little conscious attention from us. Giving conscious attention to them may save us from feelings of boredom. Unfortunately, it cannot make the job anything other than it is. However, doing the washing up, for instance, with attention to what we are doing and how we are doing it, i.e. not pulling ourselves out of shape to do it, will result not only in cleaner dishes, but also avoidance of the results of pulling down.

DRIFTING OFF

When we do something requiring little attention, if we don't consciously maintain what attention is required, or consciously take up and direct some other activity, we will drift off. It doesn't matter what the job is. For instance, teachers marking maths answers by rote from an answer crib may miss that the answer in the crib is nonsense and mark right answers wrong.

When we drift off, we may continue on 'automatic pilot', but like an automaton we may not notice changes, which ought to cause us to modify what we are doing. This can lead to unsatisfactory results in some circumstances and danger in others.

DRIFTING OFF IN THE DRIVER'S SEAT

We all need to be aware of the dangers of 'drifting off' when driving the same journey day in day out. How often have you been 'somewhere else altogether' for a lot of your daily commute? Every now and then somebody doesn't notice that the lights have changed and an accident happens. How often might it have been you? Use the procedures in this book to keep you safe from harm.

Perhaps the most pernicious thing about drifting off is that we have trained ourselves to do it. How could we have done such a stupid thing? Let's start with school ... It is well known that school can be a severe trial for some children. Not all children are very good at schoolwork and, though they may start off by trying hard to understand, if success doesn't come fairly quickly, any point in making an effort to pay attention soon eludes a child – he or she can feel doomed to failure. Fear of failure carries with it unpleasant feelings, which can be avoided by drifting off. Contrarily, failure may not be due to being a 'dumbo', it may be due to ignorance and that ignorance may be due to drifting off from boredom initiated by the child not being stretched and losing interest.

Adult life too is full of empty periods. Waiting for, sitting on, standing up in buses and trains. Waiting in traffic jams. Waiting at the dentist's, at the doctor's, in the supermarket queue. We can try to read on the train or bus, but someone else having a chat can render any attempt at purposeful activity hopeless. At those times, when the present moment is not very interesting, or not very demanding, or sometimes because life is too demanding, there will be a tendency to drift off. It's the desire to drift off, the choosing to drift off, which is such a problem to us. Especially when it is a habit.

> The message is clear. Lying down for up to twenty minutes
> is a glorious opportunity for drifting off. It is also a glorious
> opportunity to learn how to stop doing it.

In the beginning, the real problem is that we are unaware that
we have drifted off. The key is recognising that you are about to
go.

Overcoming drifting off

No amount of effort will make any difference. Trying to 'do' something will make it worse. The answer is straightforward, but you
will have to be prepared to give it time and be prepared for 'failure', especially in the beginning.

One method for overcoming drifting off is to actively engage
the mind in the present moment. Explore the room with your eyes
insofar as you can, that is, without moving your head.

> Always keep your eyes in focus, all the time you are lying
> down. If you close your eyes to do the 'staying in the here
> and now', you will drift off.

Listen. Be aware of the scents on the air. What can you taste? Be
aware of the touch of your clothes and the pressure of the floor.
What's the temperature? Do you register a flow of air? Do these
activities without adding a commentary. To start up an interior
monologue is to drift off.

Then 'explore' yourself with your *full attention* and keep your eyes
open! Give your attention to each part of your body in turn – be
aware of where it is in space. Start with the head, and the jaw, then
the neck, the torso (chest, back, belly), legs, feet, hands, arms. Then
be aware of yourself as an entire body in space. (You have really good
feedback being flat on your back on a firm surface.) You may have to
do this by first being aware of the head, then, maintaining your
awareness of the head, move on to the neck. Then, move on to the
torso, and so on, until you are aware of your whole self.

WHAT TO DO IF YOU NOTICE YOU ARE NOT LETTING GO

During your 'tour', you may have registered some muscular contraction, somewhere that hasn't quite let go. Or you may have felt or thought you did. It is vital you understand that if your muscles are contracting, it is because of some electrical impulse from your brain. *Your muscles* connect only to *your brain*.

If we feel something is tight, we usually experience a desire to do something to free it up. If you do 'do' something, what is likely is that you will contract a muscle in opposition (which is the only thing you can 'do'), the most likely result of that being that the contracted muscle(s) will contract more! But the tightness is only there because we are doing something already. The electrical impulses from our brain are causing our muscles to contract. Therefore, if muscles we do not want to contract are contracting, what we must do is ... stop sending the electrical impulses.

We have three sorts of muscles: the heart, involuntary muscles (like those in arteries or the wall of the intestine) and voluntary muscles. The voluntary muscles are the ones we usually think of as muscles: we can feel them with our hand, see them move, or see the effect of their movement. When we want to move, we don't usually think in terms of muscles at all.

Supposing I want to scratch my head ... All I need to think is, 'I want my hand to go from wherever it is now to just above the point that's itching.' Then if I extend my fingers and move the tips back and forth with the right amount of vigour, my head will be being scratched. Actually, the things we do most often seem to take place as if they were reflexes. My head itches and I am scratching it. We did, though, learn how to do these things once upon a time. But because it was such a long time ago, they appear to be 'automatic'. If our acts truly were automatic, then we would really be stuck with them. If it was the itching head that automatically caused the scratching, we would scratch every time it itched, regardless of the effect. We know that scratching things can make them sore and sometimes the more you scratch, the more you itch. If it were automatic, we wouldn't be able to stop even if the scratching was damaging us. However, the truth is that our voluntary acts are voluntary however much of a habit they are. The fact that they were learned (chosen), means that we can unlearn ('unchoose') them. Your head itches but you don't have to scratch it. You can say 'no'.

> *The first thing to do is do nothing*

So, to return to lying down ... If we think we detect some contraction somewhere the first thing to do is do nothing.

Our habit is to *do something*, our habit makes us *feel* compelled to do something. It's only a feeling. Do nothing and the feeling will go away.

The feeling of compulsion is characteristic of habit. We have to consent before any habitual activity takes place. What we must learn is to separate the habit from the consent.

Suppose we have noticed that our jaw feels tight. Are our teeth touching or even being pressed together? If yes, then the jaw is probably tight. When relaxed, our lips form a seal against the outside world. Our teeth are there to be used for eating, they don't need to be pressed together unless we are eating. Having decided that our jaw is tight we remember:

1. not to do anything
2. our brain is making our jaw tight
3. this is a voluntary movement

So, just as at some level in the brain, we have decided to tighten our jaw ('grit our teeth'), we now give it our attention and consciously want it to let go. This means giving attention to the actual physical part of us, not just to the words in our head or the idea of it. In fact, if we give our attention to the jaw there need be no words, nothing but wanting this bit of us, which occupies that part of our body in space, to let go. That is what should then happen.

But what if it doesn't?

First, you didn't just want it to be free, you did something. Second, you didn't really have your attention on the body part, you were reciting words; or you were thinking the idea but not giving your attention to the jaw at the same time. Third, the tight jaw is a bit of a bigger pattern of tightening. Fourth, the cause of this tightening, or the bigger pattern, is because, at this moment, you are thinking about something that is habitually associated with tightening the jaw.

The 'cure' for the first and second is to go through the process again. And again and again. Let's look at the third. Suppose that one of your constant habits is to screw the face up. Tightening the jaw would almost certainly be a part of that pattern. If you just want the jaw to be free without freeing the other tensions in the face, the jaw can't undo because you are maintaining a habitual pattern that requires it to be tight. So, in order to get the jaw free, you must want the face to let go as well. Don't *do* anything. Give your attention to your face and jaw and want them to be free. The more particular you can be, the more successful will be the outcome. Are you pursing the lips? Want them to be free. Are you screwing up the face around the eyes? Want it to let go. Are you wrinkling your forehead? Want it to become smooth. Whatever you detect as part of this 'pattern', want it to let go.

Finally, the fourth. Are you maintaining a pattern of thinking that is causing you to tighten the jaw (and, no doubt, screw up the face)? Supposing that you have just been carved up by someone who was driving with utter disregard for the safety of others. You have had to brake violently and swerve sharply to avoid an accident. In the first place, you will probably react by feeling fear and pulling yourself more out of shape than usual. As the fear subsides it may become replaced by seething anger and a desire to get even. You get home in one piece, but your ordinary everyday pulling out of shape has been made much worse. You decide to lie down on your books before things get worse, and someone gets short shrift because you're out of sorts with yourself. You go through the procedure (this takes your mind off what has just happened) and the initial moments of lying down. Now, you are going through the procedure, outlined above, but at the same time the incident is still hovering around the edges of your consciousness. All the time you are thinking, 'There might have been a crash', you will be continuing the muscular contraction that goes with the fear, the anxiety and the anger.

In choosing to think and feel those things, you are choosing to pull yourself out of shape.

You will not be able to let the jaw go unless you let the thought go. If you cannot let the thought go, then you must think about it in a practical way. There wasn't a crash, no one was hurt. If you cannot think about it practically, then think about something else, deliberately turn the pulling out of shape thought aside. In this case, going through the procedure for lying down once more would be a good idea.

If you cannot do either of these things, then you must realise that is because you don't want to. If you don't want to stop, then you won't stop. If you don't stop, you will pull yourself out of shape. Get up. Go and do something practical. In other words, give your attention to something else. You have to *think* different thoughts to *do* something different.

HOW DO HABITS INFORM OUR THINKING?

Just as habit gives us a sense of compulsion to do something, we sometimes feel we are compelled to think certain thoughts. That it isn't possible to change our minds. That if we let go of these particular thoughts, we would be betraying ourselves, or letting down someone or something. If, though, convinced of its rightness and its necessity, we follow a reasoned course of action that goes against our normal way of thinking about a particular subject, we sometimes feel 'bad' about it.

If this is the case, the uncomfortable feelings are likely to be the result of the habitual pattern of bodily behaviour that corresponds with the thoughts. The thinking is habitual too. For instance, if someone does us a 'bad turn', are we the sort of person that won't rest until we have got even? Or do we put it down to 'bad luck', to being in the wrong place at the wrong time, nothing personal, let it go? With our general casts of mind goes our own particular muscular patterns. In a situation that excites a particular mental attitude, it is very difficult to act against type.

If the person is a 'get even' type, then it may be several weeks (and sometimes years) before they let an incident go. All the time it is 'on their mind' (even if it isn't conscious), they will be pulling themselves out of shape because of it. The question we must ask ourselves is where does the 'type', the predisposition, come from?

We are born, of course, with some hereditary influences. It does not make any sense from an evolutionary point of view that those influences should be a straitjacket. Just because we are, say, disposed to lose our tempers more quickly than another person does not mean that we are condemned to lose our temper quickly or, indeed, that we need ever lose it. What it means is that we have a greater problem to solve in terms of what is appropriate social behaviour than someone who has a 'longer fuse'. Doesn't having a 'short fuse' really mean that when things don't go our way, our predisposition is to view the world as a non-amenable place? The child that displays temper has not yet developed a mature enough understanding of the world, has not understood that when things are not going his way the answer is not to abandon all control. He does not stop, think and try another approach. He or she merely thinks that a display of tremendous energy will make some difference, however inappropriately applied or directed.

Most of our patterns of behaviour are laid down in childhood.

If the object of the child's aggression is a person and the person somehow manages to give the child the impression that this behaviour is successful, then the child is led to believe that this is a viable way of being in the world. It is a 'successful' behaviour that the child will repeat in similar circumstances. (Not to mention trying it out in others.) Yes, we're back to habit again.

Free will

The American philosopher William James gave a very practical definition of free will. He considered free will the ability to think the thought you choose to think. Being able to do so means ridding ourselves of our habitual ways of thinking (because if we don't we will continue to think the thoughts we always think). If you are one of those people who find taking decisions difficult, you will appreciate that this is not as easy as it sounds.

We can't change our behaviour just by changing our mind. Even if we can think whatever we want to think, we behave in the way our habit dictates.

HOW LONG SHOULD I LIE DOWN FOR, HOW OFTEN AND WHEN?

Sometimes it feels as if it would be good to stay lying down for ever. Falling asleep on a headrest made up of books once will convince us that this is just another misleading feeling.

Obviously it takes time for things to lengthen out and we want to make the most of the straightening out that is going on. To that end we want to lie down for as long as we can, for up to a maximum of twenty minutes. Even if you could only lie down for one minute, it would be worth doing, for there is much for you to get out of just going through the lying down procedure. One minute will not allow time for much straightening, but most of the shutting down of muscular contraction will have happened. If you are going to lie down only once in the day, then try to get as close to the maximum twenty minutes as possible.

If you are going to be able to lie down more often, say six times a day, then obviously 6 x 20 mins = 2 hours is a considerable chunk of the day. Let's consider the good times to lie down and see how that affects things.

The first is fairly soon after getting up in the morning. Wash and dress first. Have breakfast. Do these two things first in order to make sure that you are awake. The reason that this is a good time for the lying down procedure is because it is so easy to pull ourselves out of shape when we are in bed. If we don't get straight before we start, we risk the whole day being dominated by pulling out of shape. You may not think that getting up twenty minutes earlier is worth it, but what about ten or five? It will really pay good dividends. Start with what you think you can manage in terms of time – you may soon find that the benefits make an earlier start worth the effort.

Some people find it more convenient, and have the opportunity, to lie down as soon as they get to work. Or it may be a good idea, if you are at home during the day, to wait until the children or other members of the family are settled.

Remembering that an aspect of lying down is to stop the headlong rush of the day and to give you a rest, mid-morning is obviously a good second time to stop. This may be difficult time for many people and I expect that, for most people, twenty minutes at this time of day would be out of the question. If it's possible though, then five minutes lying down is a lot better than nothing.

The third time is fairly obvious: the lunch break. If you can do it, ten to twenty minutes lying down will really help you through the rest of the working day. It's cheaper than browsing the shops, too!

The fourth time to suggest itself is afternoon tea time. It may not be possible if you are out at work. But it is a very good time for those with home responsibilities to get themselves set up for the early evening rush.

The fifth time is important if you want to get something out of the rest of the evening. Go through the procedure as soon as possible after coming home from work. Or, if you are at home, at some convenient time between, say, 5.30 p.m and 7.00 p.m.

1. Wash and change first.
2. Eat a snack and get a drink if you need to.
3. 1 and 2 done, the sooner you lie down, the better. If you can make it twenty minutes, then that's great.

This will really set you up for the evening. Even if that is an evening of watching your favourite television. It is worth moving your evening meal a little later so that you can do the lying down procedure before you eat. Hence, the snack. Lying down when you are hungry is an unnecessary and an unproductive penance. If you are going out straight from work, then see if you can find some way of lying down first.

The sixth time is just before you go to bed. You will get better rest if you get into bed being straighter and it will help you not pull yourself out of shape so much during the night. However, don't wait until your eyes are closing. You do not want to fall asleep on your books for a couple of hours. Many people should go to bed sooner than they do. Let this new routine help you do it.

Of these times, the three that are most convenient for most people are a) as soon as possible in the morning; b) shortly before going to bed at night; c) between 5.30 and 7.00 p.m. If you can only make the time to lie down once during the day then I strongly suggest it is option c). Try to lie down for the maximum twenty minutes. The next best time, if you can manage it, is lunchtime. In the end, these times can only be a guide and an indication of what you might achieve. After all, you may be a shift worker or a night worker and then they simply do not apply. Therefore, the general rule must be lie down at least once a day for up to twenty minutes, preferably at a time when you think that you can get the most benefit.

PRACTICAL PROCEDURE 2

GETTING UP FROM THE FLOOR

Do not do a sit-up.

You could roll on to your side and reverse the procedure for lying down. There is, though, a better procedure.

You are going to roll over so that you end up on your hands and knees. You need to have sufficient space to your left or right to do this. Decide whether you are going to roll to the right or the left.

- Look to that side by letting the eyes lead the movement and let the head follow.
- Let the movement of the head follow immediately the eyes begin the movement. Do not tilt the head back.
- The head should still be on the books but now resting on its side.

Gaze at the floor at shoulder level and put the back of the hand of the side to which you have turned, somewhere on that line.

- The arm may be completely extended or it may be bent at the elbow and is going to act as a roll bar.
- Return the head to its former position, leading the movement with the eyes and letting the head follow. Do not let the head tilt back.

You are going to roll around your long axis. That is, as if you had a pole that went straight through the top of your head and came out at the other end of your torso.

- Begin the roll by looking to the side with your eyes, letting the head follow, continuing the movement through the neck, through the torso, into the hips and lastly the knees.

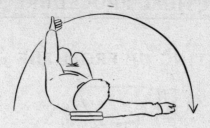

- Do not sit up. If you go hips or knees first, you will twist the back.

This movement will not have sufficient momentum to succeed by itself, so you will use your other arm to increase it.

- As you begin the rolling movement with the eyes and head, use your free arm to increase the energy of the roll by throwing the hand, with some vigour, to the place it will be when you are on your hands and knees.
- This hand is now about two feet further on than the resting hand but in the line of the shoulders.
- From the turn of the eyes through to being on the hands and knees, the pattern is one continuous sequence of movement.

This may seem difficult to do. It isn't, but you do need a complete idea of what you are aiming to achieve. You must not straighten the legs as you do it. The most important thing of all is having the intention to end up on your hands and knees.

If the procedure doesn't quite work, get onto your hands and knees anyway and think about why it went wrong. (Straightening the legs, insufficient intention and sitting up are the usual reasons.) Resolve not to do whatever it was next time.

Assuming that you are now on your hands and knees, the gaze of the eyes should be at the floor underneath your shoulders. Do not drop the neck forward. You are now going to get up from the hands and knees position. On the bottom of the pelvis are two very bony lumps. One on each side. These have the technical name of ischial tuberosities. Because they are the lumps of bone we are meant to sit on we shall call them the sitting bones.

- Send the sitting bones towards the ankles and let the torso follow.

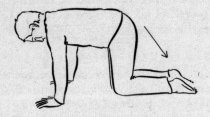

- Allow the torso to come into the upright.
- Do not tilt the head backwards. You should be gazing at the floor just in front of your knees.

Next we are going to move to the 'kneeling up' position.

- Look up to see where your head will be when you are kneeling up. Start this movement with the eyes and let the head follow – as before.
- Return the head to its previous position.
- Send the head to its position above the knees and let the torso follow so that you are now kneeling up.

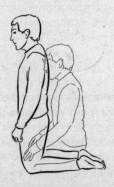

Some people find sitting back on the ankles tough going. If you are one of those, then you need to combine two activities and let them flow on one after the other.

- Send the sitting bones back towards the ankles.
- A tiny bit before they get there, send the head to its position above the knees. (You will have to guess where the head ought to go. After you have done it a couple of times, this will not be a problem.)

The next step is to get onto one knee. (Space considerations may well make it necessary to move one leg rather than the other but otherwise either leg will do.) The object is to place the foot of the leg you have decided to move just in front of the place that the knee was.

- Send the foot of the leg you have decided to move out to the side (away from the centre) sweeping the lower leg over the carpet.
- Very rapidly after, send the knee forward in an upward arc.

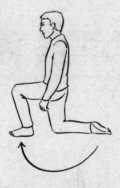

- Place the foot on the floor just in front of the knees. (The rotation that's necessary for this takes place in the hip joint.) You should now be 'kneeling up' but on one knee and one foot.
- Without tilting it backwards, send the head straight up to the ceiling and let the torso follow. You are now standing up.

Stand still for a few moments to allow for any adjustment that the body needs to make because of the change to standing up. Unless you don't need to use your 'lying down' space for something else, now is the time to pick the books up from the floor. Falling over them in the dark, for instance, will not be a happy experience. Use the same procedure as you used to put them down (p. 56).

PRACTICAL PROCEDURE 3

BEING UPRIGHT – STANDING

Now is as good a time as any to consider the problem of being upright with good use.

When you get up from lying down, the first thing you may notice is that you want to adopt your habitual upright stance. This will usually include the following activities:

- pulling the head backwards and down on the neck so that you are now looking at the horizon (this may also involve pulling the neck diagonally forward and down)
- arching the lower back (this usually involves raising the rib cage forward and upwards towards the ceiling; it also may be experienced as thrusting the hips forward and there will be a forward rotation of the pelvis)
- bracing the knees (this is actually quite a complex movement, however, the result of it is that the knees come backwards under the body, and inwards towards each other, making the leg stiff)
- tightening the front of the ankles (the effect of tightening the ankles and bracing the knees is to lock the legs into rigid pillars)

It is a common delusion that it is necessary to stiffen the legs in order to remain upright. As already mentioned, the support function of the leg is the result of a dynamic interaction between the calf muscles and the ilio-psoas muscles. The muscles, which lead to the knees being braced and the front of the ankles being stiffened, do not need to work at all for you to remain upright. When the leg is in the braced state, the joints of the leg, including the hip joint, are being pushed into each other. This makes movement difficult.

You may be standing with your feet too close together with either too small or too large an angle between them. You may also be clenching your teeth, pushing on the inside of your mouth with your tongue, screwing up your face, forming fists with your hands, bracing the arms, raising the shoulders. If you notice any of these things, want them to let go.

- Let the jaw fall so that just the lips are touching. There is no need to purse them.
- Let the tongue lie flat in the bottom of the mouth.
- Let your cheeks go and let your forehead be flat, i.e. stop wrinkling it. (If it is wrinkled give it a vigorous rub with your hand.)
- Let the hands go and the arms hang by your sides.
- Let your shoulders come down.

Improving the upright stance is a little more difficult and may have to be done before you can achieve any of the above.

IMPROVING THE POSITION OF THE HEAD

Another common delusion is that the neck muscles have to work to support the head. As if it would fall off if they didn't. It won't. What we want is to find a neutral resting position for the head. This position exists when the eyes, resting naturally in their orbits (sockets), are gazing at the floor three to four feet in front of the ankles. It is also the position in which the big muscles of the neck cease to work and the head is held in a position of balance by the ligaments on the back of the head.

Fortunately for us, the muscles that move the eyes are independent of the rest of the muscular system. This means we can achieve the neutral poised state of the head in the following way:

- if you are not looking at the floor about three to four feet in front of your ankles, then lower the gaze of the eyes
- immediately you begin to lower the gaze, let the head follow the movement so that all the time the eyes are in a neutral position in their orbits
- do not drop the neck forward

If you try to pull your head into position, you will make things worse. As soon as you start to look down your own nose, stop and start again. It means that the head was not following the movement. If you get the same result again, it probably means that this is the best that you can do for now and the situation may improve when other adjustments occur. Let the gaze be as low as it can with the eyes resting naturally in their orbits. (Fist test p. 63.)

A NOTE ON RESTING THE EYES NATURALLY IN THEIR ORBITS

If you have trouble with the procedure above, I suggest the following, which I have borrowed from Bates' Method of eye improvement. I believe it is called 'palming'.*

Raise your hands and place the palms over your closed eyes, right to right and left to left. Do not press with the hands but allow the eyeballs to rest on the palms. Do not try to see anything; you are just resting your eyes. When the eyeballs are not jumping about and there is a general experience of 'seeing' blackness, take the hands away and open the eyes. You should have let go of any untoward contraction in the muscles that move the eyeball and they ought now to be in a neutral position.

Please note: I am not in a position to recommend or condemn Bates' Method. I merely borrowed from it what was useful to me and it would be wrong not to acknowledge my source.

IMPROVING THE SITUATION OF THE FEET AND LEGS

Many people stand with their feet too close together. Each foot should be more or less under the shoulder of its own side. That is, say, at a distance of four to six inches between the heels.

Another problem is that people often stand with feet parallel. That is, the toes of both feet point in the same direction – straight forward. I know that this is a position that is adopted in Tai Chi,

---

* Palming is described in the book *Better Eyesight Without Glasses*, William H. Bates, Holt, Rinehart and Winston Inc., New York, 1943.

Karate, Aikido and no doubt many other activities. It is not, however, the natural neutral position of the foot. There is a tendency, in assuming it, to brace the knees and it needs considerable care if this position is to be adopted with good use.

We are interested in getting the natural, neutral, position of the foot. Once we have mastered that then we can learn to adopt other foot positions with good use of ourselves.

There should be an angle between the feet of about forty-five degrees. (Half a right angle.) Note that this does not mean having one foot pointing straight forward and the other pointing forty-five degrees away from it. It means splitting the angle so that one foot points away from the straight line to the same degree as the other foot.

Another common error is that people pull themselves forward over the ankles, stiffening the ankles. This means that they are constantly contracting the muscles of the front of the lower leg. No activity is required in these muscles to remain upright. In fact, contracting them when there is no need makes us contract even more the muscles of the legs that do have to work, which will result in us pulling ourselves out of shape.

It is very important for us to understand that the leg works as a whole. So that when we are merely standing, being upright, the following will happen.

- If we pull ourselves forward over the ankles, we will brace the knees back and tighten the hip joint.
- If we brace the knees back, we will pull ourselves forward over the ankles and tighten the hip joint.
- If we tighten the hip joint, we will brace the knees and pull ourselves forward of the ankles.
- Equally, if we free any one joint, all three will have to let go.

The hip joint is not one that most people are 'in touch' with. Asked to bend forward from the hips the majority of people will bend at the waist. Ask people to stop bracing their knees and they will tend to bend the knees rather than free them. The ankles, however, can be freed in much the same way as the head can, i.e. by letting go of the contraction of the muscles involved.

Before you try to do this in your standing, I would suggest that you try out the following procedure. Read the following note first.

NOTE

The whole body is constantly moving. It is always falling in and out of balance. This is because the point of perfect balance is such a fine one, and ordinary bodily activities such as the beating of the heart and breathing are constantly disturbing it. As a rule, we don't notice this movement at all. The restoration and adjustment of balance is perfectly automatic and we don't need to notice it. If, though, we start to stabilise the structure by fixing it with misuse, for example, stiffening the ankles, we interfere with this natural process. The body isn't meant to be fixed, it is meant to be free to move in any direction in a fraction of a second.

What we need to do is restore the possibility of our natural balancing act.

The exercise

Stand with your back to a wall or a closed door. Make sure that the door opens away from the side you are standing. Make sure that the backs of your heels are about four inches from the wall (or door). You may have to stand a little further away if you have a large bottom or the forward thrust of your hips makes your back lean a long way backwards.

Poise the head by lowering the gaze of the eyes. (See above, p. 96.) Maintaining the poise of the head, you must now want two things to happen at the same time.

1. You must want the whole of your body to fall backwards from the ankles as if it were a plank of wood, stood on its end, falling over. Fall until your upper back comes into contact with the wall. Let the back touch the wall, but do not lean on it.
2. You must want your sitting bones to go down and forwards towards your ankles. This is your real sitting bones going down and forward to your real ankles. Give your attention to those

parts of you. This counteracts the forward thrust of the hips.

You may feel that as soon as you touch the wall you go forward again. This is the muscles of the front of the leg doing their habitual contraction. Come back again. It may take many attempts before you can allow yourself to be 'back over the ankles'.

If you can get this right, the whole of the leg will undo:

• your hips will free
• your knees will unlock
• and you will not be thrusting the hips forward
• the body will be balanced on the ankles
• and you will not be pulling yourself forward over them

This sounds a simple enough thing to do, but you must make sure that you do not tilt the head backwards, thrust the hips forwards (making the back reach the wall too soon) or hold onto the knees, which will be trying to let go (perhaps not letting the back reach the wall at all). You will feel that you are falling a long way even though it is obvious that you are not. We tend to be afraid of falling and we will not want to let go because it feels a long way.

When you have had some success with this exercise, try it standing about a foot away from the wall. The object is only to 'fall' back as far as you were falling before. Just as far as it takes to free the ankles, not all the way to the wall. If you fall too far you will find that you will feel you want to brace your knees again. Don't. Bracing the knees will make you fall over. Standing this close to the wall you know you can't fall far, but if you tense up, move closer.

When you feel brave enough and you don't brace your knees it is a bit of fun to let yourself fall all the way back from a foot away. It makes a bit of a thump, however! Do not tilt your head backwards or you will hit it on the wall. It's more scary than you think, but if you can do it, you will have exercised your courage a little bit more and enhanced your confidence.

The next stage is to do the procedure away from the wall. Stand with the feet about six inches apart at the heels, forty-five degrees between them, adjust the poise of the head and allow yourself to come back from the ankles as you send the sitting bones down and forward to the ankles. The actual backward movement is no more than an inch (25mm). The knees will unlock and you may feel wobbly. It's only a feeling.

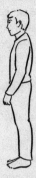

A cautionary note ... It may appear to be possible to manipulate the pelvis up and down without letting go the bracing of the knees. This will not bring about the desired result. All the joints must free for any of them to be free. You will not be doing the hip joint or lower back any good if you are bracing the knees and moving the pelvis.

STANDING FOR A LONG TIME

Standing in one place

This is not something that we do very well. Our feet do not respond well to constant pressure. We tend to stiffen the legs – even after we have learned not to. This being the case, the ideal solution is not to do it at all. However, sometimes standing still in one place is forced upon us.

One way of dealing with it is to stand with the feet quite wide apart, say a foot between the heels, feet angled as before. This widening of the base reduces the influence of the natural swaying of the body mentioned previously. This position can be maintained without stiffening the ankles or bracing the knees but there is already a tendency, anatomically, to fix the hip joint simply because of the width of the stance. Also, this stance is quite difficult to move from. (More on this when we talk about taking a step and walking.) It is very important with the side to side stance to make sure that the weight is even on both feet. It is very common to see people leaning on one hip; it is also easy to see the pulling out of shape that goes with it. Keeping the weight even on the feet overcomes this.

However, if you maintain the poise of the head and come back from the ankles as you send the sitting bones down and forward to the ankles, you should be able to stand without too much discomfort for some time.

A better way of standing in one place involves widening the base of the stance but front to back and not side to side. From a balanced and poised standing position, take a step forward, or back, with one foot or the other. If you are tall, your front foot may well be a little in advance of your back foot. For the rest of us, if the toes of the back foot are about level with the ankle of the front foot, the base is wide enough. The angle between the feet should be forty-five degrees and the weight should be evenly on both feet. This fore and aft stance does not have the anatomical

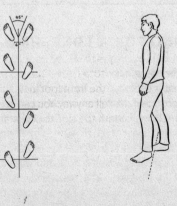

disadvantage that the widened side to side base has.

When you have to stand in one place for some time, you need to take advantage of what movement possibilities there are. These are more easily exploited in the fore and aft situation.

- Remembering that the feet to do not care for unrelieved downward pressure, take the weight alternately on to one foot and then on to the other.
- If you shift the weight onto the back foot (move the whole of you backwards over the ankles *without* tilting the head back, arching the back, or tightening the knees), you can then lift the front foot up onto the outside edges of the heel without lifting the foot from the floor.
- It will feel a little as if fluid is draining from your foot. (It isn't, it just feels like that.)
- Put the foot down and come back into the even weight position. Make sure your head is poised, the knees are free and the sitting bones are going down and forward to the ankles.
- Take the weight forward onto the front foot. (Come forward over the ankles, as a whole, don't tilt the head back, don't brace the knees, don't bend forward at the waist, don't drop the neck forward.)
- Without twisting, or bending to the side, or dropping the pelvis on one side, let the knee of the back leg go forward so that it takes the back foot right onto the toes.
- Let the foot 'drain out'.

This process is more successful when raising the front foot. Therefore, the best way is to do the front foot and then, by bringing the front foot back to the level position, advance the other foot so that it becomes the front foot in its turn. This changing of feet is good in and of itself anyway. You can see that this foot relief is difficult to achieve with the side to side stance.

FEET
- If you brace the knees, you will tend to pull the weight of your body onto the inside edge of the feet.
- It is the feet that transfer the weight of the body onto the surface you are standing on.
- The weight should be carried across the balls of the feet along the outside edge of the feet and on the heels.
- You should not notice the weight more on one part than another.
- Do not turn the feet onto their outside edges to get the effect. This will make you tighten the knees.
- Poise the head, come back from the ankles, send the sitting bones down and forward to the ankles. This will achieve the right distribution of weight.

Another problem we must think about when we are standing still in one place for a long time is the return of blood from the lower limbs to the heart. The efficient return of blood from the bottom half of the body, especially the lower leg, is dependent on leg movement. The contraction and relaxation of the muscles of the lower leg helps to pump the blood back up. You will no doubt have seen some poor soldier faint at some military pageant, having been standing still for a long time. Of course, the armed forces are aware of the problem and the soldier may or may not have been doing the exercises they were given to prevent it happening. However, the 'stand at ease' position is a braced one anyway and the 'stand easy' position is still a side to side one. The exercises they do to alleviate the problem are to sway backwards and forwards from the ankles and to over-contract and release the calf muscles. These obviously work for the majority but, unless you are bound by military discipline, you can add a much better one. You can lower the height and raise it again:

- starting from your balanced and poised position, let both knees go at the same time to lower your height (two or three inches is enough)

- without tilting the head backwards, put the head up so that you regain your standing height again
- do this several times

You are really making your muscles work to raise your body weight. They relax as soon as you reach your poised position. (It might be funny to see a military parade with the troops bobbing up and down, but we wouldn't mind if we knew why they were doing it.)

Standing but with room to move about

Even standing at bus stops and in supermarket queues we sometimes have very little room to move but often we may find that although we cannot sit down, we can move. If you are having to wait but can move, then mix standing still, as suggested above, with slowly walking backwards and forwards. If you are going to be upright for a long time with no possibility of sitting down, working in a shop, for example, or at a workbench or machine, then see if you can find something to lean on from time to time.

Leaning backwards

There are two possibilities for this:

1. Leaning against something high, a wall, for example.
2. Being able to get the back of the pelvis in contact with something.

If there is a ledge at the right height, big enough for you to get your sitting bones on and strong enough to take your weight, sit on it.

---

1. Get your back as close to the wall as you can. Do not pull yourself back from the ankles but let your weight come onto the wall. If you move your feet forward one step, the wall will really be taking quite a lot of your weight and giving your feet and legs relief. You can do the foot raising, too.

2. If there is something pelvis height, then you can get the back of the pelvis on it and let the weight come back onto the surface. The thing to be careful of here is leaning over backwards from the waist, which you must not do. If you can let the back be straight as you let the weight come back, then there is more relief to be had from this because more of the weight of the torso is being taken.

FOOTWEAR

When we are walking on a surface that gives a bit, when the foot touches down, we can probably get away without having heels on our shoes. When what we are walking on is hard, we are almost all probably best off with footwear that has some sort of heel, or is made of something that is going to take up some of the shock of impact. High heels are difficult to walk on: the foot is constantly sliding into the toe of the shoe (this can damage your toes), and they require more contraction in the calf to keep us upright (since they tip the wearer forward). When I have been asked for advice I have said that if it were necessary for me to wear them I would wear them for the shortest time that I could get away with. So, what is a 'high' heel exactly? Answer: anything much taller than an inch. It is possible to learn to wear high heels and use yourself well. However, the sliding forward in the shoe remains a problem. Obviously, the higher the heel, the greater the slide. The essence of it is to allow yourself to come as far back over the ankles into the upright as you can.

We are almost all probably best off with footwear that has some sort of heel

Platform soles … When these shoes first came out, there were many reports of people falling over and hurting themselves, even breaking ankles. This is probably the reason they disappeared from the shops. Recently they seem to have reappeared. If you want to wear them, you must always bear in mind that the sole of the foot provides us with vital information about where we are in space. It tells us that we are in contact with the floor. At least, this is what our brain makes of the information. In reality, if we are wearing shoes of some sort, we are in contact with the inside surface of the shoe. Probably, even with low-heeled, normal thickness sole shoes, it is the reason that we sometimes stumble, especially if the surface we are walking on is not truly level.

With platform soles, what the brain interprets as the floor surface may be several inches above the floor. Unless you are constantly aware of this it is very easy to stumble. Once you have stumbled, you have a weighty object at the end of your leg that is quite difficult to control. Restoring your footing is not easy and it is likelier that you will fall over than when wearing low height shoes. If you fall over you will probably hurt yourself. If you fall over when your shoe is jammed (against the floor on an uneven paving stone, say, or you do not manage to clear a kerb with the shoe), you can do very unpleasant things to your ankle. Keep this constantly in mind when you are wearing them.

PRACTICAL PROCEDURE 4

WALKING

WHICH POSITION TO START FROM

Start from the side to side stance position (i.e. heels level with each other, six inches between them, forty-five degree angle between the feet).

There are two basic considerations about walking:

• how to move in your chosen direction
• how to get the foot off the floor

HOW TO MOVE FORWARD

Obviously you have found some solution to this problem otherwise you wouldn't be able to walk forward at all. As I said earlier, most people do not start their movement by going forward but by transferring the weight to one foot by leaning to the side. This is so that they can take the other foot off the floor. (There are other variations that also pull us out of shape, like leading the movement with the hips, but the transference of weight is the same.)

Though it is important to get the foot off the floor with the best use possible, taking the foot off the floor with either good or poor use (i.e. whether or not you pull yourself out of shape to do it) does not, of itself, make you walk. You can hold the whole leg out in front of you and it will not make you overbalance. You can extend a foot out to the floor in front of you without moving the torso forward at all. You need only leave the torso vertical and put the other foot out in front of you to end up flat on your back! We move forward because it is our intention to do so. It is refining the intention, what we want to happen, which is the basis for improving our forward movement.

The good use solution

First of all, adopt your balanced and poised standing position with the normal side to side foot position. It is easier to move from this position than the fore and aft position. The reason that we don't fall forward is because of the work that the muscles of the calf are doing. If they stop working we will fall forward from the ankles. (Note. To fall backwards you have to stiffen your knees either before or after you have been pushed.)

It is possible to fall forward from the ankles without taking a step. Unless that was our intention or our feet were stuck, most of us would stick a foot out to save ourselves. Walking is not falling down and saving ourselves by sticking a foot out. The intention to walk forward causes the brain to stop telling the calf muscles to contract or, probably more likely, not to contract as much. The effect of gravity is to make us fall forward. In other words, the forward movement requires no muscular activity on our part. We need to allow ourselves to come forward over the ankles as a whole unit, as a plank of wood balancing on the ankles might fall. The head should go forward first – without tilting it backwards, of course. We will go forward as long as it is our intention to go forward.

Walking is not falling down and saving ourselves by sticking a foot out

The amount we need to go forward before we should begin to lift the foot from the floor is about a quarter of an inch. There should never be the sensation that gravity is taking over, that we really are about to fall flat on our face. Remember that your habit of standing has been to pull yourself forward over the ankles. If you don't move your foot as soon as the forward movement has begun, you will want to fix your ankles. If you try to walk with fixed ankles, you will have to lean to the side or lead with the hips to get your foot off the floor. We control the forward movement by putting our head through space without it ever losing height – carrying it evenly through the scenery, as Kip Keino, the record breaking Kenyan runner, once put it. It is very important when moving forward to have some place that you want your head to go. Be specific about where you are moving to.

I've been saying, throughout the book so far, that when the head is in the balanced position, the eyes will be gazing at the floor three to four feet in front of your ankles. If you carry on looking there, however, you won't be able to see where you are going. You do not have to tilt the head back to raise the eyes. The eyes can and should move independently of the head. To see where you are going, raise the eyes. If the head is to be tilted back, it must follow the movement of the eyes and not precede it. This will limit the opportunity for pulling your neck forward and out of shape. If you tilt the head back to move the eyes up, you will pull your neck forward. The alternative will be to stiffen the neck muscles and, in order to see the floor, 'look down your nose'. To see where you are going to put your feet, lower your gaze and if you tilted your head back, let the head follow immediately to come into the poised position. In walking forward, it is necessary both to see where you are going and to see where you are about to put your feet. Therefore the gaze of the eyes should alternate between looking forward and looking three to four feet in front of you. There is no real need to tilt your head back simply because you are walking. In moving your gaze up or down it is very important that your eyes stay in focus. This way you will see the whole of the surface you are to walk on and all the obstacles between where you are and where you are going. Letting the eyes go out of focus, remember, is a prelude to drifting off.

When walking anywhere, stay in the here and now. Do not drift off. Drifting off when you are moving about can be a serious health hazard.

Give your attention to where you're going and how you are getting there, i.e. how you are using yourself. In the unlikely event that you do not know what is between where you are standing now and what is three feet in front of you, you must explore that area by allowing the torso to come forward from the hips as a unit without tilting the head back. To come back into the vertical, you should let your knees go a little to lower your height (one inch) before bringing the torso back into the vertical. Again, without tilting the head back. Allow the leg to return to its proper length by sending the head straight up – do not tilt it back.

HOW TO GET THE FOOT OFF THE FLOOR

You may recall that the other muscles we must use if we are to remain upright are the ilio-psoas muscles. These are also the chief muscles we use to lift the foot from the floor. We do it by pulling the thigh up towards the torso. Folding the leg upward onto the body. As you do this the foot will come off the floor heel first. When the thigh reaches an angle of about forty-five degrees to the vertical, the toes will come of the floor.

Remember: you must have the intention to move your head at the same height through space all of the time you are walking. So, as the toes leave the floor, you will already be travelling forward. Bring the foot back towards the shin – do not curl your toes. At the same time, allow the lower leg to straighten so that it makes almost a straight line with the upper leg. Over-straightening it is bracing the knee while the leg is in mid-air.

There is no need to push off with the toes. Unless you have some artistic reason for the contrary, the heel ought to come into contact with the ground first.

In continuous forward movement, your heel will touch the ground because you are moving forward. In other words, you do not have to use any muscular effort to get the heel onto the ground. If you thump the floor with your heel, it is because you are pulling the lower leg backward to the thigh. It is a waste of energy, jars the whole body and doesn't do a lot for your footwear. Also, you will almost certainly be pulling yourself down towards the floor as you do it. The answer is to carry your head forward, keeping it always at its starting height. Walking forward like this will give you the normal size of your stride.

As you continue to move forward, the weight will come onto the front foot. It is important that you do not tighten and fix the ankle. As the weight comes onto the front foot, the leg becomes vertical and you will find that your back foot is already on its toes. Flex the thigh towards the torso to take the foot off the floor and extend the leg as before.

To walk more quickly, move your head forward more quickly. This really boils down to wanting your head to go *through* space more quickly. There is another way of covering the ground faster, which still depends, however, on the head leading the movement more quickly, and that is to lengthen the stride. To lengthen the stride, it is necessary to bring the thigh to a higher position before extending the leg. Do not take a stride so big that the head is no longer controlling the forward movement.

To move more slowly, want the head to go through space at a slower rate.

Our usual method of walking is habitual, a learned pattern, and because of this all aspects of it are habitual. You will find that even when you are having some success in taking the foot off the floor in a new way your stride will tend to want to remain the same. If you try to go more quickly, for instance, and try to do it directly with the legs, you will find that you fail more often than you succeed and that you go back to your old way very quickly. Leading the movement from the head will solve the problem. It is very useful to practise mixing up different stride lengths with different speed intentions. You may be amused to find that you can move very slowly taking very large strides. It really does depend on the speed at which you want your head to go forward.

PRACTISING TAKING THE FOOT OFF THE FLOOR

You may find that your habit of leaning to the side or leading forward with the hips is so strong that you want to work on picking the foot up as a practical procedure in itself.

Stand facing a wall or a closed door. (Remember not to be on the side the door opens out towards.) Be in your poised and balanced standing position with the normal foot stance about one foot from the surface of the door/wall. Place the palms of the hands on the surface at just below shoulder height. The fingers should be pointing straight up. If they are not, it is probably because you are sticking your elbows out to the side. Let the elbows fall and let the hands turn so that the fingers point up towards the ceiling.

I have divided the procedure into two parts, but there is no reason why both parts should not be worked at in one session. They are just different aspects of the same thing.

For the first part, the hands are there to give you a feeling of security. Without transferring the weight to the other foot, let one knee go forwards towards the wall.

- The direction the knee should go in is following the line of the foot – about half of forty-five degrees to the 'straight forward' line.
- The knee should go out until the foot is up on the toes.
- Do not let the hip drop.
- To get the foot back, put the heel back on the floor.
- Change legs and repeat.

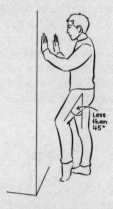

When you can do this quite well without pulling yourself out of shape, you may consider speeding the process up to a normal walking pace and sending the knee a bit higher up towards the ceiling. When the thigh reaches forty-five degrees to the vertical, the toes will come off the floor. Let the lower leg hang vertically down from the upper leg and the foot hang from the lower leg so that the toes are pointing at the floor. Place the foot back in its starting position.

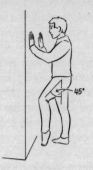

You will notice that with no intention to go forward you do not go forward just because you are taking your feet off the floor.

The second part does have intention to go forward. Stand as before with your hands on the wall. This time allow yourself to come forward as a unit from the ankles so that the weight comes onto the hands. Immediately bring the thigh up to forty-five degrees so that the foot comes off the floor. The lower leg should hang straight down from the upper leg. It should not be flexed backwards or extended forwards, and the foot should hang from the lower leg as above. Place the foot back in its starting place. Come back into the vertical by wanting the back to come back into its vertical position. This is done by extending the arms, not

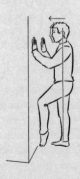

pushing on the hands. As the back goes back, the weight should come off the hands. Change legs and repeat the process.

Taking one step forward to get into the fore and aft stance

This is about half a normal step. You need to want the head to go forward for as long as it takes to get the foot off the floor and extend the leg and then stop wanting it to go forward. You should end up with both feet on the ground and the weight evenly on each foot. If more weight is on the back foot, you did not send the head forward for long enough. If more weight is on the front foot, then you kept the head going forward a little too long. It's quite subtle and for that reason alone worth working at.

To get back to where you were, i.e. to take a step back, you need to want your back to move backwards through space. Do not round the back and do not tilt the head backwards. The foot is taken from the floor in exactly the same way – the thigh comes up toward the torso – but this time, as soon as the toes leave the floor, you put the foot back beside the back foot. (About six inches apart, remember.) Let the weight even out on both feet.

Getting into the side to side stance by taking a step forward, means moving the head forward so that the weight comes onto the front foot as we bring the other foot forward to place it by the side of the front foot. Let the weight even out on both feet.

If we are standing in the fore and aft stance, or as a matter a fact in a side to side stance, which is wider than hip width apart, to bring the feet back to our hip width side to side stance is to go 'uphill' against gravity. We can exploit gravity to walk backwards from our balanced starting place by letting the back move backwards through space, but it is in moving forward from it that we really get the advantage. That is what we want to do most of anyway, isn't it?

PRACTICAL PROCEDURE 5

WALKING UP, OR CLIMBING THE STAIRS

This is different from walking along the flat. In this section of the book, I am talking about the sort of stairs we find in our houses or in buildings. Climbing stairs (the same is true of walking uphill) is the most strenuous activity that we will usually encounter during the course of our daily lives.

Let me try to give you some idea of the effort required of the body. Next time you are at the supermarket, pick up four or five 3lb bags of flour. Hold them in front of you and lift them up to the level of your face. A couple of feet say. Heavy, aren't they? Your body probably weighs at least as much as about thirty-two 3lb bags of flour, and maybe a lot more. To get from one floor of your house up to the next probably means raising yourself vertically by at least 10 feet. Let's multiply the weight of the supermarket flour by the height raised: we get a number between twenty-four and thirty. If we think about raising our body weight 10 feet, we get a number probably not much lower than 960. If lifting the flour was hard work, think how much harder it is going to be to lift yourself upstairs.

By the way, just so we don't spend our time fishing for red herrings, the number of stairs or how steep the slope is does not affect the problem. It is how much body weight there is and the vertical height we have to be lifted that matters. If we didn't have sufficient strength, we wouldn't be able get upstairs at all and some people will reach a point where they can't. However, if you can do it at all, it is possible to do it with much less stress and strain.

HOW TO DO IT

Stand correctly at the foot of the stairs. Raise the gaze of the eyes, and this time let the head follow. (Make sure it follows at once.) Look to see where your head will be when you are standing at the top of the stairs. Lower the gaze of the eyes, letting the head follow, to return your head to its poised, neutral position. The movement is going to be led by you putting your head from where it is now to the place it will be when you have reached the top of the stairs. You do not need to look any more to see where your head is going now that you know. Tilting the head back would drag you back down the stairs.

Begin the movement and immediately take a foot off the floor by sending the knee in an arc forward and upward (flexing the thigh on the torso) and place as much of it as you can on the first tread. Keep the diagonal upward movement of the head going (without tilting it back) as you pick up the back foot to place it on the next tread up and continue in this manner until you are at the top. Height is gained by the front leg extending after its foot has made contact with the tread. The necessary forward movement comes from the head. The leg will take care of itself if you can get the intention for the head right. It may be that you get a push up from the toes of the back foot, but that too will look after itself if you get the right intention for the direction of the head.

Any pulling out of shape (e.g. by pulling the head back and down, stiffening the knees, bending to one side) will tend to take you down towards the stairs and therefore make the job harder. So do not bend over, especially backwards, or twist in any way. When you have reached the top of the stairs walk away from them. Standing at the top of the stairs with your back towards them is not safe.

PRACTICAL PROCEDURE 6

WALKING DOWN THE STAIRS

It would be good if this was the simple opposite of walking up the stairs, wouldn't it? It isn't. If you were to stand at the top of the stairs and project your head forward and down to where it would be if you were standing at the bottom, you would have a very nasty accident. As a general rule, if you are standing at the edge of any sort of drop, even if it is only one step, you do not want to be swaying forward with the head leading the movement. You will fall. If you want to see what is immediately in front of you, take at least one step back before you bring your torso forward from the hips. Make sure your head does not get as far forward as the edge. If you want to look over the edge of any sort of sheer drop, get on your hands and knees, for preference, lie down. The potential for you to fall off if you are standing and your head goes in front of the edge is enormous. (Please find out that I am right about this by falling off your back doorstep before you try to prove me wrong by looking over the edge at Beachy Head.) Falling down the stairs can be as final as falling off a cliff. So we want to avoid that as well.

HOW TO DO IT

Stand poised, at the top of the stairs, with the front of your foot at the edge of the first step. Without allowing yourself to come forward, take a foot off the floor and poise it over the first tread. As soon as the foot has cleared the floor, let the knee of the other leg go out over the foot so that the leg folds up and your height is lowered. When the front foot has made contact with the tread, pick the back foot up, poise it over the next tread down and continue down the stairs. It is the ball of the foot that will come into contact with the tread first. Because the foot will be at an angle to the 'straight forward' line you should get most of your foot onto the tread even if your feet are quite big. The body should never be forward of the foot that is coming into contact with the next tread down.

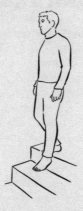

Coming downstairs and walking downhill are almost as demanding as walking up. The muscles are now acting as a brake to stop gravity getting us to the bottom very much faster than would be good for us. If you feel insecure, or are a bit 'wobbly' walking downstairs, then you should use the stair rail or place your hand on the wall for balance. The mistake people make in doing this is not getting close enough to the rail or wall before they start. If you lean, you are already taking yourself out of balance and increasing your chances of falling. Rest your hand on the wall or stair rail before you start but *do not lean* on it.

A kitchen 'step up' is a useful piece of equipment when working on improving your use in going up and down stairs. That is to say you can practise getting on it and off it as if it were a single stair away from an actual staircase. The fact that it is probably higher

> *The body should never be forward of the foot that is coming into contact with the next tread down*

than the average stair will simply make you think more about what you are doing. Place it near a wall so that you can touch the wall in case you feel insecure. (If you do, you will have pulled your head backwards and down. Lower the gaze of the eyes …) You can also try walking up the first two or three stairs and coming down them.

PRACTICAL PROCEDURE 7

SITTING DOWN IN AN UPRIGHT CHAIR

This is about getting from standing to sitting on ordinary office, kitchen or dining room chairs.

There are two components to getting into a chair: lowering the height and moving the body back through space. If you stand in front of a chair, close enough for the chair to touch the back of the legs, and you lower your height with proper use but without moving the body back through space, you will end up squatting in front of the chair. Moving backwards through space, especially if you are not taking a step, is something that we do not like to do (because we are falling) and mostly we do it badly. But if we do not let the body fall backwards, we cannot position ourselves over the chair. There are two common ways people overcome this problem. They either completely abandon themselves to gravity, or create a lot of muscular contraction, thus pulling themselves badly out of shape, as they put their sitting bones onto the chair and round over to counterbalance the effect of falling.

A BETTER WAY TO SIT

Stand in front of the chair in your poised balanced position. Your knees should not be braced. Send your back backwards, so that you are coming back over the ankles (like a plank of wood falling). Remember that bracing the knees as you move backwards will make you fall. Immediately you have begun this movement, let the knees go. At this point, you should be falling like a stone.

- As soon as you let the knees go, allow the torso to come forward from the hips.
- Do not round it over, the torso must be straight.
- Do not tilt the head back.

- The torso comes forwards so that the head is once more above the feet.
- The gaze of the eyes at this point is at the floor between your feet.

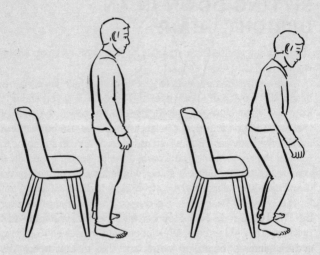

Coming down into the chair without coming forward from the hips is possible but is much more demanding. In getting the head back above the feet, you are restoring balance and are no longer falling backwards totally under the influence of gravity.

This will still have you going into the chair pretty fast. The braking mechanism is in the legs, but only the brain knows how much braking is required. If you try to do it directly, you will do too much. This is one of the reasons why people pull themselves out of shape when getting into a chair. The key to control is deciding at the outset how fast you want to fall. When you come into contact with the chair you should be on your sitting bones and forward from the hips. Allow yourself to come back into the upright by wanting the torso to hinge back at the hips. Like a door opening.

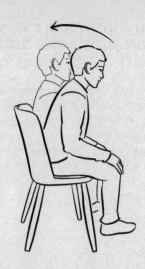

ENDING UP ON THE EDGE OF THE CHAIR

In the beginning, you may not have much control over where you end up in the chair. It depends on how far you have allowed your-self to come backwards and whether, when you come forward from the hips, the head is above the feet or out in front of them. You will become more and more skilled with practice. Be that as it may, if you are sitting too close to the edge, you are either going to slip off or create massive contraction in the legs in trying to stay there. If you are too close to the edge, fold your hands lightly into fists, place the knuckles on the sides of the chair further back than your bottom. Put the head back up towards the position it would be in if you were standing. (Do not tilt the head back.) If it helps to extend the arms, do so, but remember that the move-ment *must* be led from the head. When you have cleared the chair, allow yourself to come back to sit on your sitting bones with your bottom between your fists. You should now be in the centre of the chair or toward the back of it.

You can do this as many times as is necessary. Once usually does it. Never wriggle yourself back.

WHERE YOU SHOULD SIT IN THE CHAIR DEPENDS ON HOW LONG YOU ARE GOING TO SIT

If you are going to be sitting for only a few minutes, then you do not need to be far back in the chair. If you are going to be sitting for up to twenty minutes, then you are going to be better off sitting in the centre of the chair. If you are going to be there for more than twenty minutes, you should be sitting right at the back of the chair so that the chair can support the weight of the back.

PRACTICAL PROCEDURE 8

SITTING IN AN UPRIGHT CHAIR

There are three major points to consider:

- which bit of us we are sitting on
- what we are doing with our feet and legs
- whether or not we are going to use the back of the chair

WHICH BIT OF US ARE WE SITTING ON?

Well, we ought to be sitting on our sitting bones, but that is often not the case. We either sit forward so that the weight is on the top of our legs, or we sit back so that we come onto the softer part of our bottom. Unfortunately, both of these things require that we misuse ourselves. I suppose that one of the reasons for this might be that sitting on our sitting bones is uncomfortable after a short while. If so, you should use a cushion rather than pull yourself out of shape.

The main reason for this misuse, however, is that we are creating a lot of muscular contraction in our legs, pulling us forward and encouraging our torso into a rounded over shape. Many people disguise the 'C' shape they have when they are sitting down by rolling back onto the softer part of their bottom.

We ought to sit on our sitting bones. This is because it means the pelvis is in such a position that the bones which make up the spine (the vertebrae) sit one on top of another, making the straightest line it is possible for them to make. Coming close to needing very little muscular work to keep it erect.

WHAT ARE WE DOING WITH OUR LEGS AND FEET?

Let's put it another way, what ought we to be doing with them? Answer: you do not need to contract any leg muscles to sit in a chair. (And if you do, you need to get rid of the chair!) In other words, even when sitting on a hard wooden kitchen chair, your legs can be perfectly relaxed. The further back you sit in the chair, the less weight will be being transmitted to the floor by the feet. So, even sitting in an ordinary chair can be a good way of getting a rest.

> *Even sitting in an ordinary chair can be a good way of getting a rest*

The main position of the legs and feet that will achieve this end is when the feet are in contact with the floor and there is a right angle at the knee.

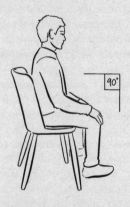

If your feet don't reach the floor when you are sitting in an ordinary chair, there are two things to do.

1. If it is a chair you don't sit on very often, just let the lower legs and feet hang. Don't scrunch up forward to get your feet on the floor.
2. If it's a chair you use all the time, say at home or at work, then

make a small platform (get someone else to make it if necessary) to put under your feet. It needs to be high enough so that when you sit in the chair your feet are flat on the platform, with the thigh horizontal and an angle of ninety degrees at the knee. It needs to be strong enough for you to stand on when you are getting into and out of the chair. You will be so glad you did this. It is something that people who worked in offices not so many years ago, typists, for instance, knew about.

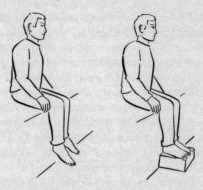

You can have one foot in front of the straight leg and, provided that both feet remain on the floor, you can have an angle greater than a right angle at the knee for both legs at the same time. If you have to sit for a long time, it is useful to be able to change the position of the feet in this way.

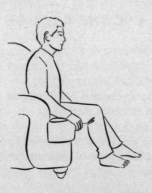

What you do not want to do is have your legs so extended that the feet come onto the heels. Even worse is crossing the ankles. Both of these tend to pull you forward so that the weight comes off the sitting bones and onto the thighs. It will only be moments before you start tightening the legs and rounding yourself over, or, alternatively, collapsing the back into the back of the chair.

Even worse is crossing the ankles

Something that is not usually done well is bringing the feet back towards the chair. We need to learn to do this in order to get out of the chair with proper use and, if you can do it well, it provides an alternative position for the foot for those 'long sits'. The critical thing is that when you have brought the foot back you must consciously let go of the muscular contraction you needed to bring it back. Do this by wanting the weight of the foot to go onto the floor. Lengthening the toes out also helps. (Give your attention to that actual physical part of you. Don't try to push the foot onto the floor.) If you don't let the contraction go, you will soon find that your calf muscles have started to contract in opposition and you are pressing your foot on the floor. It will not be long before you are pulling your torso round. Then you will have to tilt your head back and you will have really pulled yourself out of shape. Getting both feet on their toes and tucked underneath the chair is even worse.

SHALL I USE THE BACK OF THE CHAIR?

Yes, unless you are sitting for just a minute or two. You *must* use it if you will be sitting for longer than twenty minutes. It is painfully obvious as you look around you, and don't forget yourself in this, that sitting up in chairs is not something that most people do well. There is no doubt that it becomes very tiring, especially if you are using your arms to work at some task. Yet we can learn to do it well for short periods and it is helpful for us to be able to do it with proper use. Some of the things we will have to sit on will have no backs.

We have considered the necessary position of the legs and feet if we are to be able to sit on our sitting bones. Now we need to consider what things we shouldn't do with our torso. When people do get the legs in the correct position, are sitting on their sitting bones and are not rounding over forwards, they still want to lean backwards. They sometimes brace themselves backwards with their hands in their lap as they do the 'sitting up straight'. Since they are now falling over backwards, the front thigh muscles work like mad to stop it happening. This is felt as a great strain. The real reason for the leaning back is that the neck is habitually carried forward of where it should be and hence being upright makes it feel as if the head will fall off backwards.

Sitting up straight is what happens when we get the set-up for it right and stop doing all the things that get in the way of it happening.

If we use the back of the chair, we can avoid many of these problems. We must be on our sitting bones even though we are going to use the chair back. If the back of the chair is to be of any use to us, we must get ourselves right back onto the seat so that when we are on our sitting bones the back of the pelvis is touching the back of the chair. Having got into this position, we then allow ourselves to fall back into the chair without leaning over backwards or tilting the head back. Let the back of the chair take your weight. Do not pull yourself back on to it. Many modern chairs have low backs that tempt us to lean over backwards where the top edge touches the back. Ideally, the back of a chair should not slope back very much and should come up to the level of the sitter's shoulder blades.

My favourite work chair is an old oak dining room chair from the 1930s. It cost me only a few pounds, but I had to re-web and re-cover the bottom. Its back is just over 21 inches long and 15 inches wide. I've been using it for twenty years. (Just to complete the statistics, the seat is 18 inches from the floor, 18 inches at its widest part and 15 inches front to back.) There are long-backed office chairs to be had now, with adjustable seat height, but they cost much more than a few pounds.

(Ideal seat height is linked to the height of the surface you are working at. You may buy a low chair that allows you to get your feet on the floor only to find that you are now sitting too low at the work surface. There is no 'magic' furniture. Furniture cannot rid you of poor use of your bodily machinery. There is no reason why you should not, perhaps by the addition of a cushion, or with a box for your feet, sit comfortably on a whole range of perfectly normal looking chairs. Including an otherwise serviceable chair that leaves you low to your work surface. The problem you have is pulling yourself out of shape habitually, due to the habitual electrical signals your brain sends your body. Unless you change, in principle, the way you use yourself so that you do not pull yourself out of shape on a habitual basis, you will pull yourself out of shape no matter how expensive the furniture is.)

PRACTICAL PROCEDURE 9

STRAIGHTENING OUT IN THE CHAIR

This isn't as easy as lying down but it will work. Use it in combination with lying down, if you can lie down.

Many people are quite rounded over, but because the rounding over process has usually taken place over a period of years, they do not notice it. When people are standing up it is often not such a pronounced feature. Even when it is obvious to an observer that someone is 'round shouldered', the person themselves, even if you show them in a mirror, will very often not accept that they are. This is because they are used to looking at the shape they have slowly become.

Get someone to sit on their sitting bones on a chair and the C shape is impossible to disguise. The head will be down towards the chest and they will be gazing at the floor space between their feet. The reason people are this shape is because they are over-contracting the muscles of the legs. So, if you can sit in the chair on your sitting bones and allow the chair and the floor to take the weight of the legs, the legs can stop contracting – after all, they no longer have to hold you up. If the legs stop contracting, you stop pulling yourself round and down.

If this is your habitual shape, there is no real reason why your brain should suddenly decide to straighten you up, so we must encourage it. As a matter of fact, in teaching, it has sometimes happened that taking a pupil onto the sitting bones and encouraging them to free the legs (by giving their attention to that physical bit of them and wanting it to be free) has resulted in them straightening out spontaneously. My experience is that this is the exception, though. You need to understand that the muscles that straighten the back out are not the same muscles that maintain it in the upright and it is these straightening out muscles that need to be encouraged. If we know what it is that we want to happen then the brain will sort out which muscles need to be used, provided that we can get our habitual way of doing things out of the way.

You are unlikely to have got into a habit with regard to the next thing to do, so with that and your newly free legs you should be on to a winner … The problem that we are trying to overcome is that our back is rounded over, allowing our head to be in the wrong place. What we want is for our head to be in the right place, which is sitting in balance at the top of our straightened out back-bone. What we are going to do is put our head where it should be. This is how we are going to do it …

- Sit in a chair on your sitting bones with your legs free. (Throughout the whole of this procedure you must keep your attention on wanting your legs to be free – letting the chair take the weight of the thigh, and letting the rest of the weight of the leg go onto the foot.)
- Do not press down onto the chair or onto the foot. (Once you stop contracting the muscles of the leg – which, while you are sitting, no longer need to work – gravity will do the rest.)
- You should have followed the procedure for poising the head which, if you are rounded over, means that you are looking at the floor space between your feet. (Fist test, p. 63.)
- Place the palm of your left hand on your left cheek with the fingers of the hand pointing straight up towards the top of the head – or as near as you can get to it. The thumb can be in front of or behind the ear; it depends on the shape and size of your hand. In the same way, place the right hand on the right cheek.
- Allow the weight of the head to come into your hands – it's heavy – but do not let the head get any lower. All you need is the desire to support the head where it is in space now. (Remember that the legs must be free all the time. If you contract them, you will pull the head into the hands and that's no good. It may feel the same as taking the weight of it, though. The question is are you contracting the leg muscles? Not 'what does it feels like?' Letting the weight of the head be taken by the arms significantly changes the situation.)
- Without tilting the head back, put the head diagonally backwards and up to the place in space where it should be. (You

must realise that there is no way you can lift your own head back into place. If you try to do that, you will end up leaning over backwards without straightening your back out. Or you will brace the legs and start to pull yourself further round and down. You must not have any desire to do it directly by muscular effort. You must take the weight of the head and you must want it to go to where it should be. As in 'I really want this heavy lump in my hands to move diagonally backwards and up from where it is in space now to where I want this heavy lump to be in space.')

- It is not the hands lifting the head but the back muscles straightening the back that moves the head. If you try either to lift the head or straighten the back directly your old habits of use will defeat you.

If this works first time, then well and good. The chances are you try to do it and stiffen the legs, or you try to do it and brace the back up, or tilt your head back. Therefore, have a rest by letting your torso come back from the hips until your back touches the chair. Give it a moment, then come forward onto your sitting bones and go through the procedure again.

Remember always that what you want to happen would happen if only you didn't do all of the things that prevent it from happening, or at the very least make it much harder for it to happen. What you are battling against is your own habitual way of doing things. You are not going to overcome your habits in an instant. You will overcome them if you stick at it and learn what you do that stops it from happening. You will then learn how to let those things go and keep them that way as you direct the new thing to happen. As I said before, the method and the time it takes are all that is required. Don't waste your time on things that can't work.

> *What you want to happen would happen if only you didn't do all of the things that prevent it from happening*

CAUTION ...

If you are elderly and rounded over, or you have a named, diagnosed condition, which results in being rounded over, or you have been fixed, surgically, in a rounded over position, it is even more vital that you take note and do not try to force anything to happen. Forcing something to happen will hurt you. It is good for you to be on your sitting bones, it is good for you to take the weight of the head in your hands and support it, but any permanent good effect and any straightening can only come through time. What we may be seeking under these conditions is not making anything better but slowing down its deterioration.

SITTING IN CHAIRS

This is something we're not very good at ... Having learned to get into a chair and how to sit in it, the next question that follows is 'how long is it good to sit down for?' The answer is 'not very long'. Whatever people may want to argue about which things we do 'naturally', sitting in chairs isn't one of them. You may be able to make a case for sitting on the floor, lying on the floor, even squatting being natural, but sitting in chairs, no. Chairs are a very recent feature in human life – only three thousand years old, if that. They are difficult to get into with good use and difficult to get out of with good use.

The human frame, however it came to be the way it is, does not endure being static for very long. Its obvious strength is in its ability to change shape and direction very quickly. Because we lead such 'stationary' lives in the modern world, we have learned to pull the body out of shape to accommodate being still. We sit in one place at the school desk, at the supermarket checkout, behind the wheel, in the office, in the easy chair. When we sit for a long time, say longer than half an hour, even when we are sitting with the best use we can muster, and using the chair for support, we tend to sink downwards and, to prevent that, fix our joints, especially the hips and other leg joints.

Take a two-hour car journey, even with good seats, and the spryest of us stiffen up. We get out of the car and want to stretch and straighten ourselves out. It is because we have fixed our joints. You will know from your own experience and from observing others that, unless we 'collapse in on ourselves' and become inert, enforced idleness can make us very restless. It is not so bad for the driver on local journeys because there is quite a lot of movement in operating the pedals, signals and steering wheel, but after one hour on a major highway at steady speed, the driver will be in much the same state as the passengers.

Sitting on long-haul buses, making lengthy rail journeys and flying can be excruciating. Bad air, no control over the temperature, dehydration, inconsiderate fellow members of the public (and their children), uncivil staff, disgruntled customers, inconsiderate bosses and work-mates, noise, vibration, etc all add to the discomfort of life, but the worst of all of these is enforced stillness. We hated it as children and most people only learn to endure it by pulling themselves out of shape.

I was pleased to read some advice given by my son's school about how to study. Quite sensibly, it said take a break every thirty minutes or so. I can't help wondering why, if they recognise this as being a good idea, they insist on keeping the children sat still in lessons for at least an hour at a time. I work for myself. When I work at my desk or at the computer, about every thirty minutes I get up and look out of the window or go and look for something, or walk up and down the stairs a couple of times, and give myself a two or three minute break. I am able to do it because of my circumstances. Try to find a way of building a short break into your work pattern. Every two hours, I take a longer break and, apart from filling the kettle, I walk up and down and above all remain standing up.

What is vital, even if you have been sitting for only half an hour, is that when you start to move, you begin by moving slowly. (I

If you can, stand up for ten minutes

am taking it for granted, for the moment, that you are using what you can of the procedures you have been learning.) As you free up, you can start to move more quickly. Unless it is an emergency, let your joints dictate the pace.

Confined spaces are difficult to sit in because it is almost impossible to get relief from a change of foot position. When this is combined with obstacles to taking a break, you can become very miserable indeed, for example, the inside seat on a crowded train or bus, on an aeroplane, or in the midst of a row of seats in the centre of a 'jumbo' jet. There is no doubt that having a bit more room to move the limbs helps. If you are in an aisle seat, you may be able to stand up every now and then. If you can, stand up for ten minutes. If possible, walk up and down.

If you are making a really long journey, where you have no control over the surroundings, you must do the best you can to survive. Part of that may be a compromise between your comfort and convenience and that of your travelling companions. On a plane the best thing is to put the seat back and your feet up, even though it may inconvenience the person behind. On even quite short journeys you are, at the very least, going to be subjected to noise and vibration, and being constantly bombarded with new visual input is tiring, especially when it is moving rapidly. All of these things are stressful stimuli and we will want to pull ourselves out of shape in response to them. I know of no way other of dealing with vibration but to acknowledge that it is a stimulus to pull myself out of shape and consciously not respond to it. Noise can be dealt with by wearing earplugs. On long-haul flights you can also listen your way through the in-flight services reducing the apparently incessant roar of the engines. I have found that trying to listen to a personal cassette or CD-player on an aeroplane is impossible; the engine noise is just too loud. Travel in front of the engines if you can afford it – you'll also get more leg-room. It is also true of trains that you get more leg-room in first class.

We have much more control over what we look at. We can read, we can close our eyes, we can look out of the window, we can watch the in-flight movie. On a long flight we will probably want to do all of these things. The thing is not to do anything different with our eyes, such as trying to see in order to pay attention. If we want to focus our eyes, that is the only decision we need to take. The rest is quite automatic. Lack of focus either means you are tired, bored or your eyes are not working as they should. Close your eyes and rest, watch something else, put your glasses on.

Our eyes will get sore if the atmosphere is too dry. Close your eyes for a bit, that will moisten them naturally. Moisten a tissue or clean handkerchief and hold it over the eyes. If you can get to the toilet area, rinse them in bottled still water.

Dehydration is another, not so obvious, unpleasant stimulus. We do not need to travel very long by any means of transport for dehydration to set in. We are very largely made up of water. In the water are dissolved salts of different kinds, including what we normally recognise as salt, sodium chloride. There is a very strict relationship between the amount of dissolved salts and the amount of water. If we pass too much water out of our body, the salts become too concentrated. We are always passing out water from the body. When it is not being replenished, our mouth becomes dry because the body has stopped automatically keeping it moist. Unlike camels, we cannot store up water in advance of need. If you drink more than your body needs at that moment, it will soon come out again. Bear in mind that you will become dehydrated and make sure that you take in water at regular intervals. This probably means taking water with you.

> *Make sure that you take in water at regular intervals*

The longer the journey, the more you are going to need. Remember to keep your coffee tea and alcohol intake at a low level. All of these make water pass out of the body more quickly than it should, and increase the effect of dehydration.

How to occupy your mind

One of the most difficult problems to deal with on a long journey is tedium. It certainly makes us pull ourselves out of shape. Watch any bored child. Even when we are driving and are meant to be attending closely to what we are doing, we get tired of doing it. Remembering that the noise, vibration and rapid visual input of the journey are tiring you, and therefore making it more difficult to attend, adding boredom to the list means the chances of you drifting off, when driving for a long time, are very high.

Just as I have suggested in the section on lying down, whilst the circumstances are ideal for drifting off – sitting seems to make the time pass more quickly. Sitting in a car, train or plane is also an ideal situation in which to ensure that you are letting the seat take the weight of the body and that you are not pulling yourself out of shape. Spend at least ten minutes every hour doing this. Refer to p. 95 for the details.

Even so, unless you are asleep, get up and go to the loo every two hours or so, and try to stay on your feet a bit. Even if you don't want the loo, there isn't anywhere else to go on an aeroplane (you can comb your hair or something). Pick a time when there is a queue so that you can stand in it. Fellow passengers realise that if you are in an inside seat, you are going to have to move every now and then. Though your visits may become tedious for them, you are actually doing them a favour in making them move.

> *Above all, do not wriggle. If you get fidgety, get up*

On really long journeys, when you're not doing the driving or flying, find a modestly challenging five-hundred page novel or narrative history or popular biography to take with you. It helps to give you a break from the more serious work of sitting with good use you may have to do, and extend the period of time over which you can do it. Above all, do not wriggle. If you get fidgety, get up. If you cannot do anything else, work at staying in the here and now.

PRACTICAL PROCEDURE 10

GETTING OUT OF THE CHAIR

After climbing the stairs, getting out of a chair is the most strenuous thing that we have to do. You have to lift your body (minus the lower legs) against the force of gravity to bring yourself upright. I sometimes think we would all be better off with those chairs that some arthritis sufferers use: a motor slowly tilts the seat towards the vertical, thus standing the sitter up. If you are neither very elderly nor extremely overweight, you will be able to get out of a chair through the use of your own muscles.

One of the greatest drawbacks for people learning how to do this properly is that they have such wrong ideas about what is involved. Those wrong ideas are embodied in habits of use. I know that this is true for every activity that you are trying to change, but the idea of getting out of a chair is a very powerful stimulus to do unnecessary and wrong things that make getting out of a chair much harder than it already is. Ranking equal with the belief that the knees need to be locked, if we are to remain upright, is the idea that one must push against the floor to get out of a chair.

Pushing against the floor is a very peculiar notion indeed. I would like you to think for a moment about which set of muscles you would need to contract to make this happen ... The calf muscles pull the foot onto the floor when we are standing up, but if you contract them when you are sitting in the chair you will get no appreciable 'push'. The muscles at the front of the lower leg pull the foot off the floor. The muscles at the back of the upper leg pull the foot back towards the chair. The muscles of your bottom lift you a little bit up in the air when you contract them ... which leaves us with the big muscles at the front of the upper leg. Indeed, it is these muscles which you must contract if you want the sensation of the foot pressing on the floor. When you do it, though, you may also notice that they push you backward in the chair. The real problem is that in thinking of pushing down you are thinking in the wrong way entirely. You must not think of pushing down but of being extended upwards. Again, knowing where you want your head to be when you are standing up is critical.

In climbing the stairs, we wanted the head to go to where it would be if we were standing on the top stair. When we are getting out of a chair, we want our head to go from where it is now above our sitting bones to where it will be above our feet when we are standing up. How is this to be done? In reality, all there is to it is putting your head from where it is now to where you want it to be – if you can *not* do all of the other things that you have learned to do and which get in the way. The real problem is learning to recognise all of those things and how not to do them. In the meantime, you get out of the chair with the best use you can.

What you need to understand quite clearly is what needs to happen mechanically. As you put your head from where it is when you are sitting, the lower leg will be stabilised to make a lower fixed point. This enables those very powerful muscles at the front of the upper leg to contract, not to pull the feet onto the floor but to raise the thigh bone into a vertical position. As the weight of the torso comes over onto the feet, there will of course be a thrust (a push if you like) between the feet and the floor.

Now, if the thigh muscles alone worked, you would end up standing with your torso horizontal, parallel to the floor. So something else must happen. Those long muscles of the back need to pull the back into the upright. This works best when the legs are not quite straight. In other words, we don't want the straightening of the back to wait until the legs are completely straight. This is best brought about by wanting the head to move diagonally, forward and up, to its position over the feet.

You must be clear that, in order to get out of the chair, two things and only two things need to happen. The upper leg is straightened on the lower leg and the torso is straightened on the upper leg. If those two things do not happen, you will not get out of the chair whatever else you do. Why do the 'whatever else', when all it does is make it more difficult for the two necessary things to happen? But before you get out of the chair, you must prepare the best position of the legs and feet for doing it.

Unless you are sitting in the middle or towards the front edge of

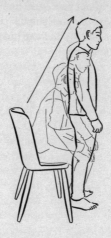

the chair, you are going to have to move yourself forward a bit so that you are. This is more or less the opposite of moving back in the chair. Place your hands on the outer sides of the chair at about the mid-point of the seat. Send your head to where you would want it to be if you were standing up, at the same time straightening up the arms and sitting yourself forward in the chair between your hands. The next thing is to move your feet. You want your feet to be in the fore and aft position with the whole of each foot on the floor. If you are too far forward in the chair you may find that your legs are too folded up and you want to contract them so it may be that you have to move one foot forward and one foot back.

It will take you a long time to learn how to do this, therefore take every opportunity you can to work on it. You stand up many times in the course of a week. Several hundred perhaps. If you do not take a decision to change the way you stand up, every time there is a stimulus to stand up you will do it in your old pulling out of shape way. Therefore, you must decide that every time you are going to stand up you will stop and set the situation up properly so that you can go through the new procedure. You have no idea what a lot of good you will do yourself by mastering it.

Stop, set it up properly, put your head from where it is now to where it will be when you are standing up, don't do any of the things that you have learned are more than what is needed. Above all, *don't tilt your head back*.

PRACTICAL PROCEDURE 11

GETTING OUT OF AN EASY CHAIR

The problem with this position is that, more often than not, your bottom will be at a lower position than the knee. Mechanically, this is a very difficult position for the body. If you have been sitting in the armchair or sofa, as we have been discussing, your back will be resting against the back of the chair and you will be sinking into the soft upholstery. The first thing to do is move forward onto the harder edge at the front of the chair. Bring the torso forward from the hip so that it is vertical (without rounding the back or tilting the head back). Move your feet a little further away from the chair if possible. Place the hands on the arms, behind you is best, or behind you on the seat. Come forward from the hips (as before) and with your arms push yourself towards the front edge of the chair. Sit on the hard edge. (I have not included a special note on how to sit in armchairs because it is essentially the same as sitting in an ordinary chair, except that you need to lower your height more. This, of course, makes it much harder to get up, since you have a greater height to lift yourself through and the thighs are at the wrong angle for the front leg muscles to be able to pull effectively – sloping backwards and down.)

In order to get out of the chair, we must get the thighs horizontal. Allow the torso to fall right forward at the hips (do not round over, do not tilt the head back) until you are looking at the floor in front of your feet. This brings the thighs into the horizontal position. Extend the thigh on the leg (as described on pg 140) to take you up as you bring the torso back into the vertical. What you are doing, in effect, is throwing yourself forward out of the chair and allowing the mechanism for making you upright to kick in at the appropriate time.

If you are elderly or very heavy, you may want to put your hands on the front edge of the chair so that when the thighs become horizontal and begin to move upwards, you can straighten the arms to get extra lift.

PRACTICAL PROCEDURE 12

LOWERING THE HEIGHT

There are many things that we do every day for which we have to be lower than our full standing height. The most common way of achieving this end is to round the back over. The back can be rounded over without pulling yourself out of shape, but it is difficult to learn to do this. Most people don't do it with good use; they do it by pulling themselves round and forward. As we have discussed, this isn't good for you, and even if you were doing it with good use there would be an overwhelming reason for not doing it. When the back comes forward from the hips without rounding over, the big back muscles support it (the same ones that straighten the back). They can support the back until it is horizontal. If we let the head get any nearer to the floor, the back will round over anyway. If the back is rounded over with good use, it is getting no help from the big muscles of the back and therefore is vulnerable to damage. Do *not lift anything in this position*.

It makes sense to find some other way of lowering our height that does not involve us in pulling ourselves out of shape or making ourselves liable to injury. We have already come across it. It is what you had to do to get into the chair. Getting into the chair has the added complication of coming backwards through space far enough in order to be able to be over the seat.

For many things it is sufficient to be in our normal poised standing position and just let the knees go only as much as is necessary to allow the torso to come forward to keep the position of the head above the feet. Signing a cheque or credit card slip at the supermarket checkout would come into this category. Once it is necessary to lower the height more than a few inches, for example, when the cashier puts the slip onto the conveyor belt, you will need to widen the distance between the feet. Don't make it too wide. (Remember, the wider apart the feet, the tighter the hip joints become.) If you are required to lower the height by any greater distance, you might be better off going onto one or both knees.

We have already discussed how the muscles of the back work to support the back when it comes forward from the hips and the head is further forward than the feet. This can be combined with lowering the height to enable us to do a variety of jobs: things like washing our face in the bathroom basin, doing the washing up, preparing food, reaching for something on the far side of the desk. Hair washing often causes people a problem. If you are going to do it over a basin, you are going to have to get quite low and get your head over the basin, which means standing back from it. You could try sitting down and coming forward from the hips. At the hairdresser's this is preferable to having the back of your neck wedged into a cleft in a basin and the head going backwards. At home, wash your hair in the shower, if you can, and if not use a mixer hose to wash it whilst kneeling in the bath.

Hair washing often causes people a problem

You can also lower the height when in the feet fore and aft position; sometimes it is essential that you do this.

What is vital is that once you have lowered the height you do not do more work with the knees than is necessary – if you do, you will lock them. You must continuously let the knees go out over the toes, allowing yourself to fall, and simultaneously, and constantly, send your head back to where it has come from. This leads to a position of being 'suspended' in space: the perpetual falling is balanced by the muscles working perpetually to take you back into the standing position. Not only does it prevent the locking of the knees but also provides a beautifully balanced isometric exercise. When you come up from having lowered your height, you must, especially if the head is forward of the foot position, lower the height a little more to get the pelvis into a good position for the back muscles to pull from.

PRACTICAL PROCEDURE 13

THINKING ABOUT USING THE HANDS AND ARMS

Almost everyone directs the use of their arms and hands in the wrong way. It doesn't happen merely because of the habits we have developed over the years. We often have a misconception about the arms. Their main function is to connect the hands to the body. Of course, we can use our arms for lifting burdens, cradling babies and so on, but that doesn't alter the case. The arms allow us to use our hands at a variety of distances away from the body in front of us and, to a lesser extent, we can even use our hands behind our backs. When we are not using the arms, they should just hang at our sides. Only a tiny amount of muscular work is needed to support them and this is achieved by holding the collarbones up.

The muscles of the arms may need to be strong, but this is only so that our hands may throw a discus, undo a tight nut, take hold of and lift a heavy weight. Most people do not realise that most of the bulk of the muscles of the forearm is made up of muscles going to the fingers. Some of them originate on the upper arm just above the elbow. (You'll see this more clearly if you grasp the forearm of one arm with the hand of the other and wiggle the fingers of the hand of the arm you are holding.)

Until very recent historical times, our hands were our chief, and most effective, way of dealing with the world. In a last resort they still are. As a general rule, all movements of the arm should be led from the hand incorporating first the forearm then the upper arm and then, if necessary, the shoulder.

If you look at the skeleton of the hand, you will see that it is not a solid lump with fingers on the end, but a collection of fingers that are separate from each other all the way from their tips to where they join the wrist bones. To give the structure solidity and to help the fingers work together as a unit they are bound together with ligaments. But they are, essentially, separate units.

That's why we can learn to type, play the piano, draw and so on.

As with everything else we do, we have to learn to use our hands and when we learn to do anything new in our first attempts, we often do too

> *Raised shoulders and tense hands are very characteristic of fear*

much. Instead of using the hand as a precision instrument, we end up tightening the hand into a fist or 'claw'. This means that instead of just moving the fingers or the whole of the hand at the wrist, say, to write or draw or use the mouse, we end up using the arm. Both raised shoulders and tense hands are very characteristic of fear and it is fear – or anxiety – that is really at the root of using our hands badly. Far too little allowance is made for different degrees of ability to manipulate our fingers and to do it at a reasonable speed. We often make speed the measure rather than allowing people the time it takes for individuals to manipulate tools accurately. We live in a society where we are meant to conform to pre-existing standards of achieving things at a certain time. If we don't, then we are compared with others who get to be considered cleverer, more skilled or 'gifted'. Of course, we want to succeed and indeed we are exhorted to try harder, encouraging us to make more muscular effort.

For a variety of reasons, many are slower on the uptake than others. I do not mean stupid. For whatever reason (which may be lack of opportunity, lack of experience, lack of background and so on), they do not quite understand what is required and haven't developed full control over their hands. (All this, of course, applies to other parts of the body.) When they appear to fail in comparison with others and are asked to try harder, the extra muscular effort they make merely gets in the way. It is not lack of effort that is the problem but lack of insight. Growth of insight takes time and input. If we are not careful, a situation is created where the anxiousness to succeed becomes constant, meaning that we are constantly tightening our hands and pulling our shoulders about.

We must learn to:
- let the hands undo
- support the arms
- lead our arm movements from the fingers or hand

Letting the hands undo

At every opportunity, without rounding over the torso, place the hands on a flat surface and extend the fingers and thumb along the surface. Do not pull the hand back at the wrist. Let go. If your hand pulls back into its usual position or you feel pressure on your fingertips, you will know that you are contracting the hand. But in order to lengthen the fingers out, you must stop contracting the muscles that pull the fingers round. Having lengthened the fingers out you can then learn not to start up the contraction that pulls them round.

Supporting the arm

If we are not doing anything with our arms, they should just hang down at our sides. Since it takes muscular work to make the palms of our hands face the front, they should be pointing backwards. If this isn't the case, don't try to do anything about it directly because what you are doing with your shoulders will be partly responsible. Getting the shoulders back into the right place is something best done through the lying down procedure (p. 53). If you are not 'lying down', then you need to develop insight into how you are pulling your shoulders around in your everyday activities and learn to stop doing it. However, if you notice that your shoulders are raised, there is no reason why you shouldn't let them *fall* back down. Do not try to pull them back down. You are holding them up. Give your attention to that physical part of you, to where the shoulders are in space, and want them to fall. It is a common thing with shoulders that you will have to go through this procedure many hundreds of times before you notice that you are about to lift them through habit and then don't.

Sitting in front of a flat surface place the hands on that surface and, without pressing, let the weight of the arm be transmitted to the surface through the hand. This will also help to lengthen out the fingers. Let the shoulders down. Then, one hand at a time, lengthen the fingers and move the hand straight up so that it is level with your shoulder – without raising the shoulders or sticking the elbow out.

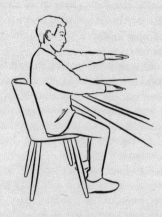

Let the hand go down to the surface again, keeping the lengthening of the fingers. If the fingers are raised up towards the ceiling, you are trying too hard to lengthen them and are, thus, over-extending them. The fingers should be flat on the surface and they should point straight forward. When you have learned how to do this, put the hand forward as far as you can (without pulling the shoulders round, twisting the hand, raising the shoulders, sticking the elbow out) and keeping the fingers lengthening. Of course, at no time are you tilting your head back. With the arm extended in front of you, want the whole arm, including the hand and fingers, to go up to the ceiling, without changing the arm position in space and without stopping lengthening the fingers. Maintain it in this situation for a few seconds. If your attention wavers, you will notice other muscles contracting. Let them go and restore your attention to what you want to happen. Bring the hand back towards the shoulder, without raising the shoulder or sticking the elbow out and keeping the lengthening of the fingers. Lower the hand to the surface. Learn to do it with both hands and arms at the same time.

Leading with the fingers or hands

If we are constantly contracting our hands, and using our shoulders badly, we will tend to lead the movement of our hands and fingers by raising the shoulder or sticking the elbows out first. Under these circumstances, the hands and fingers have become subservient to the 'connecting rods'. If we want to do something with our fingers or hands, we must learn to move them from where they are now to where we want them to be in the most direct way possible.

Try sitting with your hands resting in your lap with the palms facing up, a good free position for the hand and arm. Touch the tip of your nose with the tip of the index finger of one of your hands. If you were leading the movement with the fingertip, it would have come straight up in front of you and the rest of the hand and the arm would have followed. The elbow would be pointing down to your thigh.

If you wanted to hold your ear lobe the fingers should move from where they are in the lap in a diagonal direction directly to the lobe. The elbow would be pointing down.

If you want to take hold of something with the whole hand, to pick up a bottle of milk for instance, extend the fingers and thumb (not so much that they bend backwards) and lead the hand with the fingertips. Let the palm come into contact with the milk bottle first, then wrap the fingers and thumb round. The back of the hand and back of the wrist should be in line. Don't form the shape of the hand before it makes contact with the object. Don't think about what you are going to do after the contact, e.g. lift the bottle, until you have made contact. When you have finished doing something with the hands, extend the fingers and then let the extension go. If you are about to tense them, let it go.

AFTERWORD

If you are like me, you have probably turned to the end of the book before you have read through what's in it. If that is the case, as far as this book is concerned, then you must now go back to the beginning, read the explanations and work through the procedures. The only thing to be gained by not working through the procedures is the knowledge that you are going to get nowhere unless you do work through them.

As I said earlier on, the example we have that we can all improve our own use on our own behalf is Alexander himself. I would not have attempted to write such a book as this unless my experience of working with small and large groups of people – indeed, working with my Training Course – had not proved to me that, provided the student works at it, a little instruction goes a long way. There is more than a little instruction in this book. I have shared with you my 'stock in trade'; I have given you insight of, and admitted you to, the instruction of the Training Course.

It is possible to have Alexander lessons for years and still not learn the Alexander Technique. Many pupils of the Technique go for lessons in order to be 'fixed', 'put right'; they turn up from time to time after they have had a course of lessons to be 'topped up'. They confuse the re-coordinating work the teacher does with the hands with the Alexander Technique. They think that the Alexander Technique is being 'done' to them. They think that they do not have to put it into practice for themselves, or that reciting a set of instructions will do the trick. There are no magic incantations. The truth is that no matter how much instruction we have, unless we as individuals put the procedures into practice in our own lives, we will not be practising, neither will we be learning, the Technique. However much help we get from others, however many Alexander lessons we have, in the end we all have to

Learning the Alexander Technique depends on the student – no one else can do the work

tread the same path that Alexander trod. Learning the Alexander Technique depends on the student of the Technique – no one else can do the work.

SUMMARY

The essence of the Technique is very easily summarised. What you do you have learned to do, and 'how' you do it is also learned. You have learned how you do what you do with misuse of the psychophysical machinery. When you do something, you want it to feel like it always does, which is confused with feeling and being 'right'. The 'how' and the 'what' and the 'feeling' are habitual. However, because you do what you do with a *misuse*, you have a general misuse of the psychophysical mechanisms on a habitual basis. You are always misusing yourself, and this is harmful to you. You need to bring about a change.

You must recognise the extra 'doing', which is not necessary, and learn to stop doing it. This will be like peeling an onion, working on one layer at a time. So, do I pull my head backwards and down and pull my neck forward? Do I raise my chest? Do I hollow my back? Do I brace my knees, tighten my jaw, clench my fists, raise my shoulders, hold my breath . . . ?

Once you recognise it, the next step is to realise that you are directing it to happen. It is not being inflicted on you by a malevolent god. Therefore, if you are directing it, you have learned to direct it – so you can learn how *not* to direct it. You can't change everything at once. Work on one thing first and, when you are having some success, add something else. But remember that you must not forget the first thing!

Recognise what you do and learn what stimulus provokes the activity in you. Here, habit actually works in your favour. Most of the stimuli we face are stereotyped, too, so if you pull your head back and clench your teeth as you walk through the factory gate, the office door, the house front door, then you know that habit says you will always do that. Here, you have isolated a stimulus that provokes this behaviour. Decide then that you will anticipate this stimulus and not respond to it in the old way.

Make the decision that:

- you will not pull your head backward and down and your neck forward, you will keep your head poised
- you will not raise the chest and hollow the back, thus shortening and narrowing it, you will want the back to be long and widened
- you will not brace your knees, you will want your knees to be free
- you will not clench your fist, you will direct your fingers to be long
- you will not tighten your jaw, you want only the lips to be touching, so let the jaw fall forward and down from the head
- you do not want to raise your shoulders, you want them to let go

The words are a means of directing your thought to that part of your body, but simply saying the words without being aware of the part of the body involved is a waste of time. You need to do both until, eventually, you will be able to dispense with the words altogether.

Your job is to stop directing the habitual thing, then the automatic mechanisms will re-coordinate you. You *cannot* 'do' the new thing. But you *can* direct it to happen.

So:

- know what you habitually do and hold it in abeyance
- formulate a clear idea of what you want to replace this habit with (always bearing in mind what you have learned about use)
- continue to hold the habitual use in abeyance whilst directing into activity your new conception. This will involve not thinking about the activity in the old way, for example, never 'sit down' again. Decide at which speed you wish to fall into the chair, come back from the ankles, let the knees go and allow yourself to come forward from the hips to bring the head back over the feet.

The whole key is for *you* to learn that you are misusing yourself, for *you* to see it. You can do this. Come on, then, back to the beginning of the book and learn how to lie on the floor. Stick at it. All it takes is following the instructions – and time.

You have my very best wishes for your success.

All Orion/Phoenix titles are available at your local bookshop or from the following address:

Mail Order Department
Littlehampton Book Services
FREEPOST BR535
Worthing, West Sussex, BN13 3BR
telephone 01903 828503, *facsimile* 01903 828802
e-mail MailOrders@lbsltd.co.uk
(Please ensure that you include full postal address details)

Payment can be made either by credit/debit card (Visa, Mastercard, Access and Switch accepted) or by sending a £ Sterling cheque or postal order made payable to *Littlehampton Book Services.*
DO NOT SEND CASH OR CURRENCY.

Please add the following to cover postage and packing

UK and BFPO:
£1.50 for the first book, and 50p for each additional book to a maximum of £3.50

Overseas and Eire:
£2.50 for the first book plus £1.00 for the second book and 50p for each additional book ordered

---

BLOCK CAPITALS PLEASE

name of cardholder _____

address of cardholder _____

delivery address
(if different from cardholder)

postcode _____   *postcode* _____

☐ I enclose my remittance for £_____

☐ please debit my Mastercard/Visa/Access/Switch (delete as appropriate)

card number   ☐☐☐☐☐☐☐☐☐☐☐☐☐☐☐☐

expiry date ☐☐☐☐   Switch issue no. ☐☐

signature _____

prices and availability are subject to change without notice